101 AMAZING USES for GARLIC

FAMILIUS

FOR MY PARKLAND COMMUNITY
#MSDSTRONG

Published by Familius LLC, www.familius.com

Familius books are available at special discounts for bulk purchases, whether for sales promotions or for family or corporate use. For more information, contact Familius Sales at 559-876-2170 or email orders@familius.com.

DISCLAIMER: The material in this book is for informational purposes only. It is not intended to be a substitute for professional medical advice, diagnosis, or treatment. Always seek the advice of your physician or other qualified healthcare provider with any questions you may have regarding a medical condition or treatment. Never disregard professional medical advice or delay in seeking it because of something you have read in this book.

Library of Congress Cataloging-in-Publication Data
2018936022

Print ISBN 9781945547911
Ebook ISBN 9781641700580

Printed in the United States of America

Edited by Lindsay Sandberg
Cover design by David Miles
Book design by Brooke Jorden and Caroline Larsen

10 9 8 7 6 5 4 3 2 1
First Edition

101 AMAZING USES for

GARLIC

PREVENT COLDS, EASE SEASICKNESS, REPAIR GLASS, AND 98 MORE!

Susan Branson

CONTENTS

16. Diphtheria
17. *Escherichia coli*
18. Esophageal Cancer
19. Gastric Cancer
20. Gout
21. Hepatitis B and C
22. High Blood Pressure
23. High Cholesterol
24. Jock Itch
25. Lead Poisoning
26. Leukemia
27. Listeriosis
28. Lung Cancer
29. Malaria
30. Multiple Myeloma
31. Nail Fungus
32. Osteoarthritis
33. Osteoporosis
34. Prostate Cancer
35. Rheumatoid Arthritis
36. Ringworm
37. *Salmonella* Poisoning
38. Scleroderma
39. Staph Infection
40. Thrush
41. Tuberculosis
42. Ulcerative Colitis
43. Vaginal Trichomoniasis
44. Vaginal Yeast Infection

CHAPTER 3: EXPUNGE PESTS | 99

CHAPTER 4: EMPLOY EXTRAORDINARY USES | 115

NOTES | 127

INTRODUCTION

GARLIC, THE BELOVED HERB

Garlic is an herb closely related to onions, chives, leeks, and shallots. It grows underground as a bulb and is covered in papery skin; the bulb is divided into sections called cloves. The cloves are creamy yellow in color, and they are the part of garlic used in cooking and for medicinal benefits. You can't mistake the odor of garlic, and once you smell it, you never forget its uniquely wonderful aroma. When chopped, minced, or puréed, the essence is strong, pungent, and spicy. When cooked, the flavor mellows and sweetens.

Garlic contains over two thousand biologically active compounds, but its flavor and aroma come from the sulfur compound alliin. This compound constitutes up to 1.15 percent of whole, fresh garlic cloves, but dried garlic can contain even higher amounts. Alliin is unstable, so as soon as the garlic clove is cut or crushed, the enzyme allinase is released from cells and acts on alliin to convert it to allicin, the odor-forming compound. The characteristic garlic odor can linger on the breath for hours. To reduce the intensity of the odor, immediately consume mint leaves, raw lettuce leaves, or raw apples.[1] These foods have chemicals that can neutralize the odor-causing compounds in garlic.

The sulfur-containing compounds and their derivatives are thought to be primarily responsible for garlic's array of biological activity, but other compounds present may also have therapeutic functions. Garlic exhibits antimicrobial, anti-inflammatory, and antioxidant activity. It improves circulation, lowers blood glucose levels, targets cancer cells, and protects the liver and nervous systems. Garlic has been and continues to be extensively researched in the hope of determining the full and far-reaching potential this herb has on human health.

THE UNIVERSAL APPEAL OF GARLIC OVER TIME

Garlic is one of the oldest cultivated plants and originated in Siberia or central Asia more than five thousand years ago. After discovery, its popularity quickly spread to different lands and cultures. Over the centuries, it was used as food, medicine, and money. It even turned up in mysticism and enchantment practices. Egyptians placed clay garlic bulbs in tombs, presumably to be used as gifts for the gods or as funds for the afterlife. This was done in the tomb of King Tutankhamen, for instance.[2] The living relished garlic, too, and used it to pay slaves building the pyramids.[3] These slaves ate the garlic, believing it gave them strength and sustenance. Not so for the upper class. They preferred to use garlic for medicinal and mystical purposes. One of the oldest Egyptian medical documents, Codex Ebers, mentions using garlic for general malaise, parasites, and circulation disorders. They also used garlic as currency. Fifteen pounds would get them a healthy male slave.

The ancient Greeks followed the Egyptian use of garlic to increase vigor, feeding it to their soldiers before going off to battle. Athletes competing in the early Olympics used it to enhance their performance.[4] Not surprisingly, Hippocrates was well aware of garlic and prescribed it to treat lung issues and abdominal growths and to detoxify the body.[5] Even though garlic was a frequent ingredient in the Greeks' diet, the smell was not tolerated everywhere. If anyone wishing to enter the temples to worship had garlic breath, they were forbidden access. The Romans adopted many Greek medical practices and continued the tradition of feeding garlic to their soldiers and sailors.[6] Dioscorides, the Romans' leading medical authority, proposed garlic be used for animal bites, joint problems, and circulatory issues.[7]

In China, garlic was a staple in their daily diet and was used as a food preservative. Chinese medicine records show an early use of garlic for mental and emotional disturbances like depression, insomnia, and fatigue.[8] Ancient Indian medicine—Ayurvedic, Unani, and Tibbi—all used garlic extensively, although the upper Brahmin classes avoided it. The lower castes, however, made full use of garlic's healing properties to treat infections and wounds and as an aphrodisiac to stimulate the libido.[9]

When garlic made its way to Europe, it was the monks who grew the herb and maintained knowledge of its therapeutic uses. Like their predecessors, garlic was given to those with physically demanding jobs in order to boost their strength and productivity. Here also the upper classes felt garlic was not fit for consumption. They may have changed their minds during the Great Plague, however, when garlic was used by many to ward off infection.[10] Doctors took to carrying around cloves to mask the smell of disease and decay.[11] The use of garlic for medicinal purposes grew over time, and it was recommended for a variety of health issues. Even the wealthy came to recognize and value garlic's benefits, despite continuing to avoid it in their diet. European folklore professes garlic to have the power to ward off the "evil eye" and was used to keep vampires at bay. To this end, garlic was carried on the person, hung over windows, and rubbed on keyholes and chimneys.

Garlic made its way to North America with the French and Portuguese explorers, although the Native Americans were already using a similar bulb that grew in the wild. Today, the fascination with garlic and its purported benefits have led researchers to attempt to validate the centuries of anecdotes and folk tales and to lend credence to the multitude of cases demonstrating garlic's healing properties.

WHAT YOU NEED TO KNOW ABOUT THE DIFFERENT FORMS OF GARLIC

When shopping for fresh garlic, choose firm, clean bulbs with intact papery skin. Make sure no mold or green sprouts are evident. Some varieties are white, while others have purple or red skin, both of which often indicate a rich flavor. Consuming fresh garlic cloves in savory dishes is a wonderful way to add flavor to food and benefit from its medicinal properties. While many people love the taste of garlic, they don't enjoy the odorous breath that follows for hours afterward. It can even seem to seep through the pores if eaten in large amounts. Raw, fresh garlic may also cause gastrointestinal upset, including indigestion and flatulence. However, if you tolerate it well and favor it as a flavoring agent in food, stock up on fresh garlic bulbs and store them in a mesh bag in a cool, dry place. They will keep for up to two months in whole form at room temperature, although lower temperatures, around 60 degrees Fahrenheit, will preserve them for close to five months. Cloves removed from the bulb will last for about ten days unless they are peeled and chopped, in which case they will remain good for up to a week in refrigerated conditions.

Garlic powder is also commonly used in cooking and is made when garlic cloves are oven-dried and ground into a powder. The powder can be sold in pill form as supplements. Most people abide by the general rule that ground spices are good for six months, but many can be kept for up to three years, especially if stored in a cool, dry place. The therapeutic benefits of garlic powder may be diminished compared to fresh garlic because the bioactive compound allicin and its derivatives are thought to be absent. The powder still contains alliin and allinase, but the ability of alliin to convert to allicin in the body has not been established. Garlic powder does, however, contain other useful components that improve health, just not the full array that fresh garlic has.

Garlic oil is made by adding garlic cloves or garlic powder to vegetable oil. This oil can be used in recipes or packaged into soft gel capsules and sold as supplements. The garlic is greatly diluted and not recommended for therapeutic purposes because of its diminished potency and high fat content. Garlic oil can be kept in the freezer for several months or in the refrigerator for four days. It should not be kept at room temperature because of botulism concerns. Garlic essential oil is made from the steam distillation of crushed, fresh garlic. It is very strong both in odor and potency, so it must be diluted. Two drops of garlic essential oil in one ounce of carrier oil is sufficient. Garlic essential oil can be used topically but should not be consumed.

Perhaps the most talked-about type of garlic for its therapeutic benefits is aged garlic. Garlic is sliced and stored for up to twenty months in stainless steel tanks containing an ethanol solution. The resulting garlic is odorless because the unstable sulfur compounds have been converted into milder ones that are said to be more beneficial and more easily absorbed by the body. This, in addition to greater antioxidant potential, results in enhanced medicinal effectiveness. Aged garlic extracts are commonly packaged into capsules and sold extensively as supplements.

HOW MUCH CAN I SAFELY TAKE?

Fresh garlic can be safely consumed on a daily basis and added liberally in food and drinks. Supplements have also proven to be safe when used as directed. Studies on garlic powder capsules have administered up to 1500 milligrams a day, aged garlic extract capsules up to 7200 milligrams a day, and garlic oil up to 500 milligrams a day without any serious side effects. All people experience bad breath, but an unlucky few may also suffer from nausea, heartburn, gas, diarrhea, or vomiting. Raw garlic applied directly to the skin can cause irritation and damage, similar to a burn. If attempting to use garlic in this way, test on a small, inconspicuous area first. When garlic is added to pastes, gels, or mouthwashes, however, this response is unusual unless the person is very sensitive or allergic to garlic. Pregnant and breastfeeding women can enjoy garlic in amounts normally found in food but should avoid higher therapeutic amounts. The same advice applies to children.

Garlic can interfere with a few of the drugs used to help control medical conditions. The absorption and utilization of isoniazid can be reduced. This is an antibiotic used in the treatment of tuberculosis. Atazanavir and saquinavir, for the treatment of HIV infection, are influenced in the same way. Medications to slow blood clotting, like warfarin, taken alongside garlic can increase the chance of bleeding. This additive effect is also a danger with antihypertensive drugs as both can lower blood pressure, increasing the risk of hypotension.

Caution must be taken when combining garlic with other herbs that slow blood clotting. These include ginger, clove, ginkgo, turmeric, and angelica. Fish oil and vitamin E also run this risk. Other products have garlic's ability to lower blood pressure, so be careful when combining garlic with cat's claw, coenzyme Q-10, and stinging nettle. Always make sure you are aware of the range of effects herbs, vitamins, and supplements have on the body to avoid unwanted and potentially dangerous events.

CHAPTER 1

ELEVATE YOUR HEALTH

HEALTH

WELLNESS

PESTS

OTHER

1. ALOPECIA AREATA (PATCHY HAIR LOSS)

Hair grows everywhere on the body except the palms of the hands and the soles of the feet. While many people spend countless hours and money trying to remove hair on the body, just as much effort is put into preserving and maintaining hair on the head. A healthy, shiny, lustrous head of hair is a sign of beauty and a point of fashion and personal expression. Hair loss is common in men and can even happen in women and children. When a person has a medical condition called alopecia areata, the hair tends to fall out in round patches. This occurs most commonly on the head but can happen anywhere on the body. It results from the immune system attacking hair follicles, causing hair loss. These follicles remain alive, however, and can later reactivate to grow hair. Each person's experience is unique, and hair loss and regrowth can be unpredictable or cyclical. There is no cure for alopecia areata. Milder forms of the disease can be treated by either stimulating hair follicles to encourage hair regrowth or preventing the immune system from attacking the follicles. People with more serious cases may choose oral or injectable medications to achieve these results, although these don't work for everyone.

One of the medications used to treat alopecia areata is betamethasone valerate. The efficacy of this drug was significantly improved when used in combination with garlic. A study including both men and women with alopecia areata observed that 95 percent of patients applying both betamethasone valerate and garlic gel to their skin saw enhanced results. After three months, the number of grown hairs increased, the number of terminal hairs decreased, and the size of bald patches was reduced. These responses were significantly better than those observed in the placebo group.[12] Mixing garlic into topical alopecia medications can reduce patchy hair loss without any additional side effects.

2. ALZHEIMER'S DISEASE

Alzheimer's disease—a form of dementia—is a progressive brain disorder that is irreversible. It can begin with greater-than-normal memory loss and result in wandering and getting lost, repeating questions, and some personality and behavioral changes. As it progresses, memory loss and confusion grow worse, and people may have trouble recognizing friends and family, carrying out multi-step tasks, or coping with new situations. In the late stage, brain tissue shrinks significantly and communication becomes difficult. Alzheimer's patients become completely dependent on others for care and often become bedridden. In most people with Alzheimer's, symptoms begin in their mid-sixties. Early onset may have genetic factors in play, and late onset arises from complex brain changes that occur over decades. Current treatment approaches encourage patients to focus on mental function and manage behavioral symptoms. Several medications have been approved by the FDA for the treatment of these symptoms.

The approved treatment options for Alzheimer's may improve symptoms but don't cure the disease. This failure warrants exploring new agents that may be effective. Garlic is one of these agents and has several compounds that are proving to lessen the symptoms of Alzheimer's and do so without inducing adverse side effects. Garlic has been shown to improve short-term memory in rats with amyloid-β (Aβ) peptides in their brain. Aβ peptides consist of the amino acids that make up a plaque in the brains of Alzheimer's patients; this plaque causes nerve cell death and the degeneration of brain function, including cognitive impairment. Various doses of aged garlic extract were orally administered to male rats for fifty-six days. They were then injected with Aβ peptide. After seven days, garlic not only improved short-term memory but reduced neuroinflammation,[13] another sign of advancing Alzheimer's disease. Aged garlic extract can prevent the deterioration of long-term memory too, as shown in an Aβ plaque–induced Alzheimer's mice model.[14]

3. ASTHMA

Asthma is a chronic condition in which the airways leading to the lungs are inflamed. When exposed to triggers (chemicals or situations that impact the body), the airways swell and produce extra mucus. The passageway for air narrows, and breathing becomes more difficult. Symptoms include coughing, shortness of breath, wheezing, and chest pain. Anyone can develop asthma, although some are genetically predisposed to it. Triggers can be allergens, from the environment or from food, or other substances like smoke, pollution, or changes in the weather. Learning what your specific triggers are goes a long way in asthma management. Doctors often prescribe controller medications like corticosteroids and long-acting beta agonists and sometimes leukotriene modifiers to help manage the condition. Short-acting beta agonists are prescribed to quickly relieve symptoms by relaxing and opening the airways.

Because of the increasing and alarming rise of asthma in children and adults, it is more important than ever to find ways to manage this condition without the overuse of controller medications. Garlic is emerging as a potential therapeutic for the regulation of asthma. One of garlic's major sulfur compounds, diallyl disulfide, was studied in a model of allergic asthma. It reduced inflammation, overproduction of mucus, and immunoglobulin E (IgE) antibody levels in the lungs.[15] IgE antibodies are produced when the body recognizes an allergen and activates the allergic response, which for asthmatics means notable narrowing of the airways. Another study demonstrated that aged garlic extract injected into the peritoneum of mice significantly decreased airway inflammation.[16] These results suggest garlic may be used to reduce airway constriction and the production of mucus to ease breathing in asthma patients.

4. ATHEROSCLEROSIS

When plaque builds up inside the arteries, atherosclerosis results. This plaque comprises cholesterol, fat, calcium, cellular waste products, and fibrin, a protein involved in blood clotting. Over time, the plaque builds up on the artery wall and hardens. The artery opening narrows, reducing the flow of oxygen-rich blood to the body. Arteries to the heart, brain, arms, legs, kidneys, or pelvis may be involved. If a piece of the plaque breaks off and is carried to another part of the body, it can get stuck in a smaller artery and cut off blood flow to that part of the body. Sometimes blood clots form on the surface of plaque and block the artery entirely at the site of the plaque. If the blockage is to the heart, a heart attack will result. If it's to the head, a stroke occurs.

Atherosclerosis can begin in childhood but most often presents itself later in life. Smoking, a sedentary lifestyle, high blood pressure, poor diet, and genetics are all risk factors that can lead to its development. Changes in lifestyle and ongoing medical care are often required to minimize damage and manage this disease.

The oxidation of low-density lipoprotein cholesterol (LDL) contributes to the development of atherosclerosis. Aged garlic extract and one of its major constituents, S-allylcysteine, significantly prevented arterial damage due to LDL oxidation and protected against cell-membrane damage and subsequent cell death.[17] Plaque volumes measured in the carotid and femoral arteries of 152 subjects determined that high-dose garlic powder intake can reduce plaque volume by up to 18 percent.[18] Healthy adults taking over 300 milligrams of standardized garlic powder for at least two years lowered age-related aortic stiffness.[19] Regular garlic consumption can help manage atherosclerosis by reducing cell damage, plaque formation, and hardening of the arteries.

5. ATHLETE'S FOOT

Wearing sandals in locker rooms and around public pools can help protect your feet from a common fungal infection known as athlete's foot. This fungus is highly contagious and can be acquired by sharing shoes, walking on infected surfaces, or touching the skin of an infected foot. Once contracted, the fungus grows on or just under the surface of the skin and thrives in moist, warm places. It's important to dry the feet well, particularly between the toes, to prevent fungus from growing. The fungi can also grow in shoes, so make sure to disinfect all footwear as well.

There are three types of infection. Toe-web type occurs between the toes, causing the skin to become itchy, scaly, dry, and cracked. Moccasin type is characterized by a sore foot followed by thickened skin on the heel or along the bottom of the foot. Vesicular athlete's foot develops as blisters under the skin. Mild infections can be treated with antifungal lotions, but more severe infections may require prescription antifungal topical medications or pills.

Ajoene, an organosulfur compound, was extracted from garlic and added to a cream to test how well it worked as an antifungal treatment in patients with athlete's foot. Seventy-nine percent of subjects were completely fungus-free after seven days of treatment. The rest of the patients were cured after an additional seven days of treatment. No recurrent infections were observed after three months.[20] Ajoene was even tested against terbinafine, an antifungal medicine commonly prescribed to treat athlete's foot. Subjects receiving a twice-daily topical application of 1 percent ajoene were cured in 100 percent of cases after sixty days of treatment, while those receiving 1 percent terbinafine saw complete elimination of the fungus in 94 percent of cases.[21] Not only is ajoene from garlic more effective than terbinafine, alcoholic extracts of garlic which contain ajoene are relatively inexpensive. Garlic can provide an effective and low-cost antifungal treatment for athlete's foot.

HEALTH

WELLNESS

PESTS

OTHER

HEALTH

WELLNESS

PESTS

OTHER

6. BEAVER FEVER

Giardia is a microscopic parasite found in soil, food, or water that has been contaminated with feces from infected animals or humans. This parasite is found worldwide, often in areas of poor sanitation, and is a common cause of waterborne illness (beaver fever) in the United States. It lurks in lakes and streams but can also be found in municipal water, hot tubs, and swimming pools. Once ingested, *Giardia* live in the intestines and cause intestinal illness resulting in cramps, bloating, nausea, and diarrhea. Infection can last for several weeks, but it is not uncommon for intestinal problems to continue for longer. Not everyone experiences symptoms, so some may pass on the parasite unknowingly. If the symptoms are severe, antibiotics can be taken to eliminate the parasite. Nausea and a metallic taste in the mouth are common side effects of the antibiotics.

When *Giardia* affects humans, it can cause nutritional deficiencies in children, weight loss, and an impaired immune system. Because it can last so long and have lingering effects, you want to eliminate the infection early.

Whole garlic extract and some of its isolated compounds, like allyl alcohol and allyl mercaptan, exhibited antigiardial activity. These components used different modes of action by changing the surface or internal structure of the parasite, debilitating its function.[22] Allicin, a major active ingredient in garlic formed when the cloves are cut or crushed, also displayed antiparasitic activity against *Giardia*.[23] Consuming cut garlic cloves may help prevent *Giardia* from infecting the body and causing sickness, or it may help speed recovery by inhibiting the parasites' viability.

7. BENIGN BREAST CONDITIONS

Some of the screening tests used to detect palpable lesions or breast tissue abnormalities are clinical breast exams, mammography, and MRI. When these abnormalities are further investigated and diagnosed as benign, they are called benign breast conditions. This term actually encompasses several different types of breast conditions: hyperplasia (an overgrowth of cells that mainly occurs inside the milk ducts), cysts (fluid-filled sacs), fibroadenomas (solid, benign tumors), and sclerosing adenosis (small breast lumps). These may look like cancer on initial screening, but a biopsy rules cancer out. Some of these conditions may cause breast pain, need surgery to fix, or increase the risk of breast cancer. Treatment is aimed at relieving symptoms.

A dietary supplement containing 150 milligrams of garlic powder and vitamins was given twice a day to patients with benign breast disease. After six months, breast pain and the palpable symptoms of breast fibromatosis (a benign breast tumor) were reduced.[24] For women considering whether to take pain medication, consuming garlic on a daily basis may be a safe and gentle way to find relief.

8. BLADDER CANCER

The balloon-shaped, hollow organ in the pelvis that stores urine after it has left the kidneys is called the bladder. It has flexible, muscular walls that contract to send urine out of the body. The cells lining these walls can mutate and grow uncontrollably, eventually forming a tumor. If left unchecked, this cancer can spread to lymph nodes or other parts of the body. Most cases are caught in the early stages and are suspected when there is blood in the urine accompanied by back or pelvic pain. Frequent and painful urination may also occur. Depending on how advanced the cancer is, surgery is often advised to remove the tumor. Sometimes the entire bladder or a small portion of it are removed at the same time. Chemotherapy drugs and radiation therapy to kill the cancer cells may be administered before or after surgery.

Garlic is a naturally occurring herb with a broad range of favorable effects that may be considered for use in the treatment or prevention of bladder cancer. It stimulates the immune system to produce compounds that detoxify carcinogens and protects against decreased immunity resulting from chemotherapy and radiation.[25] Diallyl trisulfide in garlic has been shown to suppress the migration and invasion of bladder cancer cells tested in the lab.[26] Spread of the cancer would be contained, giving the patient a higher chance of recovery. In another study, whole garlic extracts were fed to mice and resulted in significantly lower bladder tumor weights and volume compared to control mice who were not fed garlic.[27] Garlic's strong anticancer activity suggests consuming garlic or garlic supplements could be used as a complimentary therapy with traditional methods of bladder cancer treatment and can be taken as a preventative to decrease the risk of developing cancer.

9. BREAST CANCER

Breast cancer starts when cells of the breast begin to grow out of control and form a tumor. Tumors are cancerous if they grow and spread into other areas of the body. The condition is much more common in women, but men can get breast cancer too. Mammograms can help detect the cancer before symptoms begin. If not detected early, breast cancer can cause bloody discharge from the nipple or changes in the shape or texture of the breast or nipple. It can also be felt as a lump. Treatment may involve radiation, chemotherapy, or surgery.

This is the most common cancer among women, so finding new and effective therapies is critical to help increase survival rates. This is particularly important when dealing with multidrug-resistant breast cancers. Garlic may offer a new therapeutic approach. Seven stabilized derivatives of garlic's allicin were able to stop the growth of breast cancer cells, including multidrug-resistant cells.[28] This offers hope to those not responding to chemotherapy. Another stable compound, S-allylmercaptocysteine, in aged garlic extract, was also able to inhibit the growth and proliferation of breast cancer cells.[29] Regular oral consumption of garlic in the diet seems advisable and is supported by the results of an Iranian study that found high dietary consumption of garlic in women reduced the risk of breast cancer.[30]

10. BRONCHITIS

Bronchitis is a respiratory disease characterized by the inflammation of the lining of the bronchial airways of the lungs. Acute bronchitis can result from a cold or other respiratory infection that causes the mucus membranes to swell and air pathways to narrow. Chronic bronchitis is more severe and is a constant inflammation of the lining of the bronchial tubes, most often caused by smoking. People with bronchitis have coughing spells and often cough up mucus. Chest pain, fever, chills, and fatigue are other symptoms. Acute bronchitis often goes away on its own after a short time, while chronic bronchitis persists and often requires cough medicine, asthma inhalers, or antibiotics if a bacterial infection is suspected.

The viruses that cause colds in adults and children often produce mild symptoms. But sometimes the body can't fight off the virus in the initial stages of infection, and bronchitis, or a chest cold, develops. To prevent this from happening, the body's immune system needs to be functioning well. Garlic boosts the immune system and has antiviral properties. It can help prevent an irritating cold from progressing into bronchitis. People who took a garlic supplement once a day for twelve weeks during cold and flu season had significantly fewer colds, and recovered faster if infected, than those in the control group who did not take a garlic supplement.[31] To help stave off a bronchial infection or to feel well sooner, try this concoction:

GARLIC TONIC FOR RESPIRATORY INFECTIONS

6 cloves peeled and chopped garlic
4 tablespoons raw honey
2 tablespoons apple cider vinegar
4 tablespoons filtered water

1. Combine all ingredients in a lidded, airtight glass jar and shake vigorously until thoroughly mixed.
2. Take a teaspoon of the tonic every 4 hours until symptoms subside.

11. CANDIDIASIS

Candidiasis is a fungal infection caused by the yeast-like *Candida* fungus. There are over twenty species of *Candida* that can infect humans, but *Candida albicans* is the most common. These yeasts normally live on the skin and mucous membranes in people and are generally harmless. If conditions in the body shift to create an environment favorable to *Candida* overgrowth, infections of the mouth, vagina, urinary tract, skin, or stomach can set in. Most causes of *Candida* overgrowth result from certain drugs, pregnancy, bacterial infections, excess weight, or an overburdened immune system. Vaginal yeast infections, white lesions on the tongue or inner cheek, painful cracks in the skin at the corners of the mouth, or crusted skin rashes around the fingers, toes, and groin are symptoms of candidiasis.

Antifungal drugs are commonly prescribed for up to two weeks. Reducing sugar and yeast products in the diet and taking probiotics are popular complementary approaches to assist in eliminating candidiasis. Daily consumption of garlic can be added to these alternative methods. Diallyldisulphide, a sulfur compound found in garlic, caused oxidative stress to several species of *Candida* and damaged the fungal cells, limiting their viability.[32] Another compound in garlic, allicin, was compared to the prescription antifungal drug fluconazole to see how effective they were in eliminating candidiasis in mice. Both were able to damage the structural integrity of the outer surface of the fungal cells, leading to cell death, but allicin was slightly less potent than fluconazole. Allicin is suggested as a complementary therapy to be used with fluconazole in the treatment of candidiasis.[33]

12. CHAGAS DISEASE

An infection of the parasite *Trypansoma cruzi* is responsible for Chagas disease. This parasite is found in the feces of a bug commonly called the kissing bug. The kissing bug comes out at night and bites people on exposed areas of the skin as they sleep, usually on the face. After it bites, it defecates. The *Trypansoma cruzi* parasite in the feces finds its way into the host body through cuts and scratches or through the eyes and mouth. The parasite begins to multiply and circulate in the blood. Initial infection lasts about two months and is usually asymptomatic. People often do not know they are infected. Some, however, experience a purplish swelling on one of the eyelids, a skin lesion, body aches, headaches, fatigue, nausea, or swollen glands. If the infection is not treated in the initial phase, it can become a chronic infection that afflicts the heart and digestive systems. This disease occurs principally in Latin America but has moved into the United States and Canada over the past few decades. Treatment in the initial stage of infection using benznidazole, a drug proven to kill the parasite, has recently been approved by the FDA. The World Health Organization reports adverse events occurring in up to 40 percent of those treated with benznidazole and nifurtimox, another drug that is not yet approved by the FDA. It is ineffective in curing the disease in the later stages but can be used to slow the progression and decrease symptoms.

As many as seven million people worldwide have Chagas disease. While the incidence in North America is relatively low, it is rising. The recent FDA approval of benznidazole to kill the parasite in the early stage of this disease is welcome and needed. However, it may take a while for the drug to become available for use, and it will likely be costly since it's the only FDA-approved medical treatment for Chagas. For those that need help now and are looking for a natural and inexpensive way to reduce parasite viability, garlic may be the answer. Ajoene in garlic was found to inhibit the growth and proliferation of the *Trypansoma cruzi* parasite in several stages of its life cycle. It changed the intracellular membrane of the parasite, causing the cell membrane to burst and killing it.[34] It may be worthwhile to consume garlic to help prevent or treat Chagas disease.

13. COLORECTAL CANCER

Most colorectal cancers begin with the formation of polyps (abnormal growths) in the large intestine. Colorectal polyps are small clumps of cells that grow in the inner lining of the colon; they can

HEALTH

WELLNESS

PESTS

OTHER

be tubular, flat, or mushroom shaped. They are very common, and their prevalence increases with age. More than one-third of people over the age of sixty have at least one polyp. They vary in number, size, and location. The most common type is called an adenoma polyp, which has the potential to develop into cancer. The larger it is, the more likely that it will develop into cancer. Having three or more of these polyps, even if they are benign, increases the probability that future polyps will develop and be cancerous. Some heredity disorders, such as familial adenomatous polyposis (FAP), cause hundreds to thousands of polyps, usually in the teenage years. If not treated, they will very likely develop into cancer. In the early stages, the absence of symptoms is common, but as the disease progresses, patients experience changes in bowel habits, rectal bleeding, abdominal pain, fatigue, and unexplained weight loss. Like most cancers, treatment is often radiation, chemotherapy, surgery, or a combination of these.

In the United States, colorectal cancer is the third-leading cause of cancer-related deaths in women and the second-leading cause in men. Early detection greatly increases the odds of overcoming this disease, but it can go unnoticed for long periods of time. A natural product, like garlic, would provide a measure of protection. Aged garlic extract can reduce the incidence of cancer by suppressing the growth and multiplication of polyps. This was discovered in a twelve-month clinical trial in patients with colorectal polyps of the large bowel. Those patients fed high doses of aged garlic extract significantly reduced the size and number of their polyps. The control group did not fare as well and saw an increase in their polyp numbers.[35] Raw, aged, and cooked garlic are effective, and a risk reduction of 30 percent was observed across several studies.[36]

14. CYSTIC FIBROSIS

Cystic fibrosis is an inherited genetic disease that affects 30,000 people in the United States and more than 70,000 people world-wide. A defective gene changes the way salt moves in and out of cells. What results is mucus that is thick and sticky rather than thin and lubricating. This mucus builds up in the pancreas, blocking the tubes that carry digestive enzymes to the intestines. Food is not properly broken down and absorbed, and malnutrition can result. Common problems also include blocked bile ducts leading to liver problems, intestinal obstruction, and infertility in men. Perhaps the organs most affected are the lungs. Mucus clogs the airways of the lungs and traps bacteria, leading to frequent lung infections, lung damage, and eventually lung failure. To date, there is no cure, but with the advent of new medications, patients can expect to live to about forty years of age. About 90 percent of patients end up dying from obstructive lung disease. It is vitally important to have a daily treatment plan that loosens and clears the airways. Inhaled antibiotic medications can be used to help fight lung infections.

Pseudomonas aeruginosa are bacteria that frequently cause chronic lung infections in cystic fibrosis patients. When they get into the lungs, they form tight microcolonies that are resistant to antibiotic treatment. Even the host's white blood cells are ineffective against the bacterial infection. When *Pseudomonas aeruginosa* was grown in the presence of a garlic extract, the susceptibility of the bacteria to both tobramycin, an antibiotic used to treat lung infections, and the host's white blood cells was increased. Administration of garlic two days before and five days after

Pseudomonas aeruginosa infection in mice significantly decreased the bacterial numbers.[37] Consuming garlic may increase the effectiveness of the body's immune system to remove the infection and increase sensitivity of the bacteria to antibiotic treatment.

15. DIABETES

Diabetes is a disease that affects the way the body handles glucose, resulting in high levels of this sugar in the blood. There is type 1 diabetes, in which the pancreas produces little or no insulin; type 2 diabetes, in which the pancreas does produce insulin, but the body doesn't use it as well as it should; and gestational diabetes, a form of high blood sugar affecting pregnant women. Some people are genetically predisposed to diabetes, but being overweight is also a risk factor. Feelings of thirst, frequent urination, fatigue, tingling, numbness in the hands or feet, and blurry vision are all signs of diabetes. Managing diabetes involves exercising, improving diet, and monitoring blood glucose levels. For many, daily insulin injections are needed.

Garlic is effective in lowering fasting blood glucose levels. Patients with type 2 diabetes were given either garlic tablets along with metformin, an anti-diabetic medication, or placebo tablets along with metformin. After twenty-four weeks, patients consuming the garlic tablets saw a significant reduction in fasting blood glucose levels compared to the patients in the placebo group. It is also interesting that garlic was able to reduce total mean cholesterol, LDL cholesterol, and triglycerides and increase high-density lipoprotein cholesterol (HDL).[38] This is especially important in diabetics with abnormal fat levels because it decreases the risk of coronary artery disease. Garlic may be used to help manage diabetes and its associated cardiovascular complications.

16. DIPHTHERIA

Diphtheria is a serious, contagious bacterial infection caused by *Corynebacterium diphtheria.* It is most commonly transmitted through inhaling expired respiratory droplets from an infected person. The bacteria attach to the lining of the respiratory system and produce a toxin that destroys healthy tissue. A grayish layer consisting of the dead tissue coats the nose and throat, making it very difficult to breathe and swallow. These symptoms are accompanied by fever, swollen glands, sore throat, and general weakness. Some people can carry the diphtheria bacteria but not show any symptoms, but they are still contagious. The toxin can move into the bloodstream and damage the heart, nerves, and kidneys. A vaccine is available today to prevent diphtheria, and cases in North America are relatively rare. In other parts of the world that don't have access to this vaccine, however, diphtheria still affects thousands of people. If contracted, antitoxins and antibiotics are administered to stop the poison and kill the bacteria.

As a first line of defense, you should consider a diphtheria vaccine. If you choose not to vaccinate or are in an area of the world where the vaccine is not accessible, you can try an old remedy using garlic. A book published in 1918 in Chicago mentions garlic as a remedy for diphtheria. It is said to "act better than anything else heretofore recommended." A garlic clove should be kept in the mouth and occasionally scraped by the teeth to release some juice. When the clove is completely mashed, it can be swallowed and a new garlic clove put in the mouth. Approximately one garlic clove is used per hour. After several hours, the author claims the grayish layer covering the nose and throat will be removed. Fever should break and return to normal in a few hours. Because those with diphtheria cannot smell or taste garlic, this remedy may be possible for many.[39] If the bulb is too hot, however, fresh garlic juice can be mixed with a sweet liquid or jelly and held in the mouth. This method should also be repeated over several hours.

17. ESCHERICHIA COLI

Escherichia coli (*E. coli*) are bacteria that normally live in the intestines of humans and animals. Many types of *E. coli* are harmless and are important to the health of the digestive tract. Several species, however, are pathogenic and cause bloody diarrhea, urinary tract infections, anemia, or kidney failure. Contraction of *E. coli* can be made from contact with infected persons or animals or from consuming food or water containing the bacteria. *E. coli* can contaminate meat during processing, and if it is not cooked to 160 degrees Fahrenheit, it can survive and infect the consumer. Sometimes cows spread the bacteria to their milk as it passes their udders. If the milk is not pasteurized, the bacteria will continue to live and pose a threat. Even raw fruits and vegetables can have *E. coli* bacteria from contact with contaminated water or people. Three or four days after ingesting *E. coli*, food poisoning becomes evident as symptoms develop. They usually subside on their own after about a week.

It is imperative to cook meats to their proper temperatures and wash produce thoroughly to remove any traces of *E. coli*. If poisoning has occurred, you can use garlic to eradicate these bacteria. Garlic powder from aged garlic effectively killed *E. coli* after twenty-four hours of exposure, while powder from fresh garlic took only six.[40] Garlic can also work synergistically with the antibiotics gentamicin[41] and streptomycin.[42] Consuming garlic with these antibiotics should provide speedy relief from an *E. coli* infection. Fresh garlic juice added to filtered water can also be used as a produce spray on vegetables and fruit to eliminate any bacteria lurking on their surfaces. Be sure to rinse thoroughly after disinfection to remove the garlic odor.

18. ESOPHAGEAL CANCER

The long, hollow tube that runs from the throat to the stomach is the esophagus. It carries food from the mouth to the stomach for digestion. When the cells that line this tube mutate and begin to divide in an uncontrolled way, cancer of the esophagus can develop. These cells can accumulate into tumors that continue to grow and can invade nearby tissues or spread to other parts of the body. During the early stages, no symptoms are noticed. As it progresses, difficulty swallowing, unintentional weight loss, chest pain, indigestion, or hoarseness may occur. Smoking and poorly controlled long-term acid reflux are significant risk factors. Surgery is commonly performed to remove the tumor with or without chemotherapy and radiation. Side effects of these treatments include infection, bleeding, painful swallowing, or accidental damage to nearby organs.

The anticancer effects of garlic have been known for some time. Its vast array of sulfur-rich compounds is mainly responsible for these benefits. Ajoene, found in crushed garlic, inhibited proliferation and induced cell death in a line of human esophageal cancer cells.[43] Diallyl disulfide, another sulfur compound from garlic, significantly reduced esophageal cancer cell viability by preventing the cells from multiplying.[44] Consuming garlic may provide a safe and effective way to prevent esophageal cancer in high-risk patients or be used as an anticancer agent in esophageal cancer therapy.

19. GASTRIC CANCER

Gastric cancer (stomach cancer) occurs when the cells in the lining of the stomach begin to grow uncontrollably. Those cancerous cells can spread to nearby organs or to the lymph vessels and nodes, where it can be carried to other parts of the body. Stomach cancer grows slowly and tends to only show symptoms in later stages. It is more common in men and in those older than their mid-sixties. The nitrites and nitrates in processed meats have been shown to cause stomach cancer in lab animals, so it's a good idea to skip the pepperoni on pizza or the bacon with eggs. Smoking can double the risk of stomach cancer, and secondhand smoke is just as dangerous. A third common cause of stomach cancer is infection with *Helicobacter pylori* (*H. pylori*) bacteria. Most people with this infection never develop stomach cancer, but long-term infection can cause inflammation of the inner lining of the stomach, giving rise to precancerous changes. Symptoms can include nausea, vomiting, loss of appetite, a sensation of feeling full, abdominal pain, and heartburn. Conventional treatments include medications, surgery, chemotherapy, and radiation.

A number of human clinical trials have sought the effects of garlic and its constituents on gastric cancer. All doses of garlic studied reduced the risk of this cancer. Higher doses were associated with higher risk reductions.[45] A European study in nutrition found that the higher the consumption of garlic and onions, the lower the risk of gastric cancer.[46] Laboratory studies have looked at different compounds in garlic like allicin,[47] S-allylmercaptocysteine,[48] and diallyl disulphide.[49] They all impact the growth, proliferation, invasiveness, and cell viability of gastric cancer cells. To capture all the cancer-fighting compounds in garlic, try consuming fresh garlic on a daily basis.

20. GOUT

Gout is a form of arthritis that causes severe pain, tenderness, and swelling in joints, most commonly at the base of the big toe. An attack of gout can come on suddenly and happen over and over unless treated. It is caused when too much uric acid in the blood builds up to the point that uric acid crystals are formed in the joints. These crystals are sharp and needle-like and are responsible for pain, redness, and swelling. Medications are used to treat acute attacks and prevent future attacks. They include nonsteroidal anti-inflammatories, corticosteroids, and colchicine to reduce pain and inflammation. Other medications to block uric acid production or increase its removal can also be prescribed for patients in severe pain. Side effects include stomach pain, nausea, vomiting, diarrhea, mood changes, rashes, and kidney stones.

Garlic has shown to be successful in improving the symptoms of other types of arthritis, like osteoarthritis and rheumatoid arthritis. It works primarily by reducing inflammation and relieving pain. Although research is lacking on the effectiveness of garlic in easing the symptoms of gout, many people swear by its effectiveness. Garlic likely acts as an anti-inflammatory and reduces the swelling associated with gout, along with redness and pain. Chew several raw garlic cloves a day. If raw garlic is too hot for the mouth, try boiling the cloves for five minutes then drinking the water once it has cooled to a comfortable temperature. This can be repeated several times a day until the symptoms of gout have disappeared.

21. HEPATITIS B AND C

These are infections caused by the hepatitis B and C viruses. Hepatitis B is most commonly transmitted from mother to baby during birth but can also be acquired through sexual contact or from sharing syringes and needles. Most adults who contract this virus have acute hepatitis B, a short-term illness. Some will feel ill for several weeks with nausea, diarrhea, fatigue, jaundice, and abdominal pain. A small portion of adults and the majority of babies and children with the virus progress to chronic hepatitis B. This long-term illness can lead to cirrhosis and liver cancer. Acute hepatitis B has no treatment other than to make the person feel comfortable until the illness passes. Oral antiviral medications can be taken to suppress the virus in chronic cases and slow the progression of liver disease. Prevention can be achieved by taking the hepatitis B vaccine in a three- or four-dose schedule.

Hepatitis C is a viral disease that affects the liver. It is contracted through contaminated blood and can live in the body for many years before symptoms begin to appear. Most people do not know they have hepatitis C until the virus begins to damage the liver and symptoms develop like fever, nausea, diarrhea, poor appetite, fatigue, jaundice, muscle aches, and bleeding issues. About 25 percent of cases in the acute phase resolve themselves without treatment. The rest can be treated with antiviral medications to clear the virus from the system. Most cases left untreated, however, will develop into a chronic illness that can cause scarring of the liver, which impairs its function, liver cancer, or even liver failure. If the liver is too damaged or low-functioning, a liver transplant may be required. There is no vaccination for hepatitis C as there is for hepatitis B. If contracted, most people need antiviral treatment to eliminate the illness or manage their symptoms.

Diphenyl dimethyl bicarboxylate (DDB) is used as a medicine in some countries to prevent liver damage in chronic hepatitis patients. Garlic oil added to DDB works synergistically to provide superior protection to the liver and was found to be even more effective than other common hepatoprotective medicines, ursodiol and silymarin.[50] A six-week dosing study with garlic oil and DDB found that patients receiving either 150 milligrams or 300 milligrams of garlic oil a day (along with DDB) significantly reduced serum enzymes that are typically elevated in hepatitis patients with liver inflammation. This demonstrates that the garlic oil and DDB preparation had a protective effect on the liver.[51] For those suffering from chronic hepatitis B or C, garlic oil taken with hepatitis medication can slow the progression of the disease by safeguarding the liver against injury.

....

22. HIGH BLOOD PRESSURE

The force exerted against arterial walls as blood flows through them determines blood pressure. The pressure is measured in the arteries when the heart contracts (systolic) and when the heart is at rest (diastolic). It is determined by how much blood the heart pumps and the resistance it encounters as it flows through the arteries. Blood pressure sustained above 140/90 mmhg (millimeters of mercury) is considered high and is called hypertension. This condition develops slowly over time, and many people have it without knowing. It can damage blood vessels and the heart. If left untreated, it can lead to heart attack and stroke. Primary hypertension doesn't have any identifiable cause, although obesity, smoking, poor diet, lack of exercise, and high salt intake are some common risk factors. Secondary hypertension has an underlying cause and could result from drugs or certain medications, alcohol abuse, thyroid problems, or kidney issues. Hypertension responds well to changes in lifestyle. Exercising more, eating a nutrient-rich diet, reducing stress, and quitting smoking and alcohol consumption should bring blood pressure down. There are many drugs available to lower blood pressure, including thiazide diuretics to reduce blood volume, beta-blockers to slow down the heart rate, ACE inhibitors to block the action of some hormones that regulate blood pressure, and calcium channel blockers and renin inhibitors to widen the arteries. All these medications come with significant side effects like diarrhea, fatigue, dizziness, nausea, erectile dysfunction, and headaches.

Changes in lifestyle should be the first line of defense against high blood pressure. The use of natural products to lower blood pressure can also assist in safely bringing down elevated blood pressure levels. The use of garlic to control blood pressure has increased in recent years, and with good reason. Garlic has been shown to significantly lower both systolic and diastolic blood pressure in hypertensive patients,[52] reducing their reliance on medications. Patients with uncontrolled systolic hypertension significantly reduced their systolic blood pressure in just twelve weeks when 480 milligrams of aged garlic extract were consumed each day.[53] It's interesting to note that the risk of bleeding was not increased in patients also taking blood-thinning medications.[54] Talk to your doctor before combining garlic and these medications. Caution is still advised. If consuming fresh or aged garlic is not preferable, garlic powder tablets can be used with the same result on systolic blood pressure.[55]

23. HIGH CHOLESTEROL

Cholesterol is a waxy, fat-like substance found in cells. It is necessary in order for the body to make vitamin D, hormones, and bile acids that help digest food. We produce cholesterol on our own, but we also get it in saturated fat and cholesterol-laden foods. It comes in two forms: HDL (the good) and LDL (the bad). High cholesterol is when there are high levels of cholesterol in the blood, both HDL and LDL. When there is too much LDL cholesterol in the body, however, it can build up in the arteries and increase the chances of getting coronary heart disease. Plaque, which contains cholesterol, builds up inside the arteries and causes partial or full blockage, leading to narrowing and hardening of the arteries. This can lead to a heart attack or stroke. Statins are drugs commonly prescribed to lower LDL cholesterol, but taking statins can cause intestinal problems and muscle inflammation.

Cholesterol levels respond well to changes in diet. Eating foods low in saturated fats and reducing intake of animal products, which are the contributors of cholesterol in the diet, will do wonders. Consuming garlic can help improve cholesterol levels, too. Patients with coronary artery disease were administered a daily dose of garlic or placebo for three months. Those consuming garlic significantly reduced their total serum cholesterol and triglyceride levels and significantly increased their HDL cholesterol.[56]

Diabetic patients also suffer from abnormal lipid levels. Garlic plus metformin, a drug to treat type 2 diabetes, were given to a group of diabetic patients while other patients received placebo along with metformin. After twenty-four weeks, the garlic group had lower total cholesterol, lower LDL cholesterol, lower triglycerides, and higher HDL cholesterol as compared to the placebo group.[57] Garlic can safely be used alone or in combination with antidiabetic medication to manage cholesterol levels.

24. JOCK ITCH

Named for its tendency to develop in athletes, jock itch is a mildly contagious fungal infection of the groin area. It can develop when the fungus finds a warm, moist place to grow. The skin becomes reddened in the crease of the groin and often spreads outward to the inner thighs, genitals, and buttocks. The rash is characterized as itchy, dry, and scaly, with red pus-filled blisters that may ooze. It tends to be much more common in men than women and in those that sweat heavily, have diabetes, have a weakened immune system, or wear tight underwear. It is spread from direct contact, so don't share towels or clothing with an infected person. Because this is the same fungus that causes athlete's foot, take care not to spread the fungus from the groin to the foot and vice versa. Keep both areas clean and dry to prevent the fungus from thriving. Antifungal ointments, lotions, or sprays can be used to clear mild infections in a few weeks. More severe infections or recurrent cases may require stronger prescription antifungal medication.

Ajoene is a sulfur compound in garlic that has antifungal activity. Ajoene was compared to terbinafine, a common medication used to treat fungal infections of the skin. Sixty men with jock itch or athlete's foot were randomized into two treatment groups, one receiving ajoene gel and the other receiving terbinafine cream. After sixty days, the ajoene gel completely healed the fungal infection in 73 percent of the men, while the terbinafine cream was 71 percent effective.[58] Garlic provides a novel compound that can be clinically used to treat jock itch, alleviating not only the intolerable itch but the fungus itself. Try heating fresh, minced garlic gently in olive oil, and when cooled, rub the oil into the skin. This can be done several times a day until the infection clears.

25. LEAD POISONING

Lead is a heavy metal naturally found in the earth's crust and is widespread in the air, water, and even some homes due to human activities. Manufacturing processes, the burning of fossil fuels, and the use of lead-based products have all increased human exposure to this metal. Lead can be absorbed into the body upon contact and can cause irreparable harm, especially to children. Although symptoms are not usually detected until blood levels are quite high, a blood test can determine the presence of lead in the body so actions can be taken before it's too late. In children, lead affects the brain and nervous system and can cause developmental delays, learning difficulties, fatigue, irritability, weight loss, and even seizures. One of the leading ways children are exposed is through eating lead-based paint chips that can be found in older homes. Other ways include eating and drinking contaminated food and water, eating off of dishware containing lead, or eating soil. Adults are also at risk and may experience headaches, joint pain, muscle pain, memory problems, and high blood pressure. Sperm count in men may be reduced, and pregnant women may miscarry or give birth prematurely. The first step in combating lead poisoning is to remove the source of lead in the environment. This may include painting over old, lead-based paint or changing dishware to lead-free brands. For more severe cases, chelation therapy is warranted. This is an oral or injectable medication that binds with lead in the body and excretes it in the urine.

Garlic is effective in reducing blood lead levels and associated clinical symptoms. In one study, 117 workers in the car battery industry were chosen to test the efficacy of either d-penicillamine, a chelator used to rid the body of heavy metals, or garlic on improving blood lead levels. After four weeks of treatment, garlic significantly improved the symptoms of irritability, headache, decreased deep tendon reflex, and mean systolic blood pressure. D-penicillamine did not. Both, however, were comparable in their ability to significantly reduce blood lead concentrations.[59] Garlic can safely be used to remedy mild to moderate lead poisoning and related symptoms.

26. LEUKEMIA

Leukemia is a cancer of the body's blood-forming tissues. Abnormal white blood cells are produced by the bone marrow and don't function properly. They can't perform their main role of fighting infections. These cells grow and divide more rapidly and continue to live when their normal cell life cycle is over. They begin to crowd out healthy cells, and symptoms begin to develop. The exact causes are not understood, but it's thought that both genetic and environmental factors are at play. Symptoms can include fever or chills, fatigue, bone pain, frequent infections, excessive sweating at night, recurrent nosebleeds, and swollen lymph nodes. Like other cancers, chemotherapy, radiation, and medications are used to treat leukemia. Sometimes stem cell transplants are given to replace diseased bone marrow with healthy bone marrow.

Because the blood cells can no longer adequately defend the body against infection, consuming garlic, with its antimicrobial properties, can help protect the body and boost immune function. This would benefit leukemia patients by helping to provide protection against infections and allow the body to focus more energy on becoming well. A recently isolated compound derivative from garlic cloves was shown to inhibit cell growth in a human leukemia cell line, showing promise as an anticancer agent for leukemia.[60] Aged garlic extract has also shown this same effect.[61] Other compounds in garlic have been isolated and tested for their influence on leukemia cells, including diallyl disulfide[62] and ajoene.[63] Both arrest leukemia cell division, preventing further spread of the cancer.

27. LISTERIOSIS

Listeriosis is a serious infection caused by eating food contaminated with the bacteria *Listeria monocytogenes*. These bacteria are contracted by humans most commonly through deli meats, hot dogs, unpasteurized milk, and soft cheeses. Most people who come into contact with these bacteria are not seriously affected and may experience muscle aches, headaches, nausea, and diarrhea. Pregnant mothers need to be very vigilant during pregnancy because listeria can be life-threatening to the fetus and newborn baby. People with weakened immune systems are also at higher risk of developing serious or life-threatening complications. This illness usually runs its course without intervention, but in high-risk patients, antibiotics are commonly prescribed.

Chouriço de vinho is a traditional Portuguese sausage made from roughly minced meat and fat marinated for several days in wine and spices. It is then matured at low temperatures for up to four weeks. Listeria can grow in the sausage during this time and cause a health threat to consumers. It was discovered that adding either powdered garlic or fresh garlic juice to the wine-based marinade kept *Listeria* numbers in the sausage low, ensuring the safety of this product.[64] Adding garlic to recipes using food prone to *Listeria* growth can reduce bacterial numbers and prevent infection in consumers.

28. LUNG CANCER

People who smoke, breathe in secondhand smoke, are chronically exposed to environmental irritants, or have a family history of lung cancer should be concerned about this disease. Smoking is especially dangerous as the number-one cause of lung cancer and the leading cause of cancer death in the United States.

Lung cancer can occur when the cells lining the lungs become damaged. Over time, they no longer function normally and cancer can develop. There are two major types of lung cancers: small cell, a rapidly spreading cancer comprising up to 15 percent of lung cancers, and non-small cell, the most common type, afflicting about 85 percent of those with a positive diagnosis. There are few symptoms in the early stages, but as it progresses, lung cancer can cause chronic cough, wheezing, chest pain, headache, and the coughing up of blood. Treatment depends on the stage of cancer and the overall health of the individual. Chemotherapy, radiation, and surgery are common options to eradicate this disease.

A Chinese study of 865 participants discovered that raw garlic consumption is associated with a lower risk of lung cancer.[65] Several of garlic's compounds have been isolated and tested individually for their effects on lung cancer cells. Ajoene, a sulfur compound in garlic, inhibited the growth and multiplication of lung tumor cells

HEALTH

WELLNESS

PESTS

OTHER

but did not affect noncancerous lung cells,[66] suggesting that ajoene's activity is selective toward cancer cells. S-allylmercaptocysteine, a stable, water-soluble compound in aged garlic extract, was able to prevent the carcinogen benzo[a]pyrene, a principal constituent in tobacco smoke, from inducing cancerous activity in human lung cells.[67] Garlic as a whole or extracted for its active compounds are promising chemotherapeutic agents in lung cancer.

29. MALARiA

The bite of a female *Anopheles* mosquito infected with *Plasmodium* parasites transmits these parasites to humans. The parasites enter the bloodstream and travel to the liver, where they begin to multiply. Some malarial parasites remain in the liver, and others are released into the bloodstream. They infect red blood cells and continue to grow and multiply inside them. Eventually, the red blood cells are destroyed, and new daughter parasites are released. They continue the cycle by invading other red blood cells. The incubation period lasts an average of ten days, after which time the human host will begin to develop symptoms. Fever, headache, chills, sweats, fatigue, and sometimes seizures begin and can be misdiagnosed as flu, particularly in areas where malaria is uncommon.

In the United States, about 1700 cases are diagnosed each year, most often from travelers returning from countries where malaria is common. Those traveling to malaria-endemic countries should take precautions and get tested immediately if symptoms develop. If left untreated, vital organs can become damaged, and in severe cases, malaria can be fatal.

The World Health Organization recommends treatment with artemisinin (sweet wormwood)-based combination therapy (ACT). Sweet wormwood reduces the concentration of the parasite in the bloodstream within the first three days of infection, and other drugs are used to eliminate the rest. Malaria is becoming resistant to ACT treatment, however, with no alternatives to sweet wormwood available. There is a vaccine licensed for use in Europe, but it is not yet available in the United States.

Finding an alternative source to current treatments is becoming more important with the rise in drug-resistant strains of the *Plasmodium* parasite. Allicin from garlic is one of the known compounds that actively inhibits malarial infection. Laboratory studies show low concentrations of allicin prevent parasitic ability to invade host cells. A four-day oral or intravenous preparation of allicin significantly decreased the amount of parasites found in the blood of mice and increased their survival by ten days.[68]

Arteether is an antimalarial drug that can clear the parasite from 98 percent of hosts after three consecutive days of 150-milligram injections.[69] In a mouse model of malaria, a much smaller singular dose of arteether followed by three daily doses of garlic oil was administered. One hundred percent of hosts cleared the parasite, and all mice survived.[70]

30. MULTIPLE MYELOMA

Plasma cells are a type of white blood cell of the immune system that normally produce antibodies to fight germs. They are mainly found in bone marrow, the soft tissue inside some hollow bones. If

HEALTH

WELLNESS

PESTS

OTHER

these plasma cells become malignant, they grow out of control and produce a tumor in a bone. If more than one tumor is present, the disease is classified as multiple myeloma. These cancerous plasma cells crowd out healthy blood-forming cells in the bone marrow, speed up the breakdown of bone, and produce ineffectual antibodies. This can lead to anemia, increased bruising and bleeding, weak bones, increased infections, and kidney problems. Men are more likely than women to develop this disease, as are people older than sixty-five and those of African-American descent. Standard treatment includes drugs that target the destruction of cancer cells, drugs that keep bones strong, or drugs that boost the immune system. Intravenous donor antibody treatment, chemotherapy, radiation, or bone marrow transplantation are other options.

People at higher risk of developing multiple myeloma may want to consider adding garlic to their diet. A study in northwest China included 220 patients with confirmed multiple myeloma and 220 healthy controls. Those eating garlic significantly reduced their risk of developing the disease.[71] Garlic, then, can be used as a preventative measure in high-risk populations to reduce the chance of plasma cells becoming cancerous and developing into tumors.

31. NAIL FUNGUS

Fungal infections are extremely common and can infect any part of the body. When fungus targets the fingernails or toenails, white or yellow spots may begin to appear. These spots then merge to form patches and spread out. The nails become thicker, brittle, and discolored, and the edges start to crumble. The symptoms occur slowly and may eventually result in the nail detaching from the skin and falling off. Fungal infections can actually be a sign of *Candida* overgrowth in the body. *Candida albicans* is a very common fungus in humans and can grow out of control in people with weakened or compromised immune systems. The good bacteria in the gut cannot compete with candida, and a systemic invasion may begin, which can show up as a fungal infection of the nails. Over-the-counter treatments are available, but they are not always effective, and the chance of recurrence is high. Prescribed oral antifungal drugs can be used that allow new growth of the nail to be fungus-free. This is a slow process and may cause a variety of side effects, from a skin rash to liver disease. Medicated polishes and creams are used, but these can take a year to get rid of the fungus. The nail can also be surgically removed, but it grows back slowly.

An effective way to get rid of fungal infections of the nail is to use garlic. Aged garlic extract inhibited the activity of eighteen strains of *Candida albicans* in a dose-dependent manner under laboratory conditions.[72] Active compounds in the garlic extract penetrated the cellular membranes of the fungi and then destroyed the internal membranes of the organelles, resulting in cell death.[73] Applying a topical solution of garlic oil (diluted in coconut oil) to the nails can attack the fungus at the site. Consuming garlic in the diet or as a supplement can also help eliminate *Candida*. With continued use, it may prevent reoccurrence.

32. OSTEOARTHRITIS

Arthritis is the most common disability in the United States, affecting more than fifty million people. Osteoarthritis is one of the two most common types and is characterized by inflammation of the joints. The joints provide the connection between bones that allow for movement, and they are cushioned by cartilage to allow the joint to move smoothly and easily. In osteoarthritis, the cartilage breaks down and causes the inflammation. Extra fluid is produced in the joint, resulting in swelling. This disease affects many people as they age due to natural wear and tear. Heredity also plays a role, as does injury from trauma or disease. Those afflicted suffer from joints that are painful, creaky, stiff, and swollen, and their range of motion is reduced, particularly in the hands, feet, spine, hips, and knees. Reducing the stress on the joint cartilage is recommended to alleviate some of the symptoms. This involves losing weight and avoiding certain activities. The goal of treatment is to reduce pain and inflammation to allow for more comfortable movement. Medications are taken as pills, creams, gels, and even injections into the arthritic joint. Side effects of these can include gastrointestinal distress such as stomach upset, diarrhea, or ulcers.

Treatments for osteoarthritis often include anti-inflammatory compounds. Diallyl sulfide from garlic is one such compound and was shown to reduce the inflammatory response in joint tissue.[74] These results were supported by another study, a dietary analysis in a large group of twins. It revealed that high consumption of garlic protected against the development of osteoarthritis by inhibiting the expression of enzymes that degrade the cartilaginous matrix in healthy cartilage cells.[75] If suffering from osteoarthritis, add garlic to the diet to reduce swelling and joint pain.

33. OSTEoPOROSIS

Osteoporosis is a bone disease in which the body can't produce enough new bone to replace old-bone removal. The process of bone absorption and replacement happens continuously in the body, and in those with osteoporosis, bone mass decreases over time. A decrease in mass and density results in weakened bones that are more likely to break. It is more common in women than men because women have lower bone masses. Osteoporosis is known as a silent disease because it doesn't produce symptoms, and diagnosis is often made only after a bone has been broken. This disease runs in families, so if a parent or grandparent had osteoporosis, there is an increased chance the next generation will have it, too. Certain diseases and medications can also increase the likelihood of developing osteoporosis. A healthy diet sufficient in bone-producing minerals, weight-bearing exercises, and medication are recommended for management and treatment.

The stages of osteoporosis in humans can be represented by ovariectomized female rats in bone loss studies. Several of these studies found that garlic oil can suppress the breakdown of bone tissue[76] and prevent estrogen deficiency–induced bone mineral loss.[77] Garlic oil was even compared to lovastin, a statin drug that helps build bone, and 17 beta-estradiol, a powerful agent to prevent osteoporosis. Like the two prescription agents, garlic oil supplemented to a group of female rats resulted in significantly less bone loss and higher bone densities and bone mineral content than unsupplemented females.[78] It appears that garlic has phytoestrogenic-like activity and can be added to the diet of peri- and postmenopausal women to prevent bone loss and the development of osteoporosis.

34. PROSTATE CANCER

This is cancer that occurs in a man's prostate, the small gland that produces seminal fluid to nourish and transport sperm. It can begin when some cells in the prostate mutate and begin to grow and divide rapidly. They live long after normal prostate cells die, and they come together to form tumors. These tumors can grow to invade nearby tissue, or some abnormal cells can break off and spread to other parts of the body. Some prostate cancers grow slowly and remain confined to the prostate. These often require minimal treatment and monitoring. Other types can be more aggressive and spread quickly. These need more invasive treatments and usually consist of surgery, chemotherapy, radiation, or hormone therapy. Advanced cases may cause difficulty urinating, slow urine stream, blood in the semen, erectile dysfunction, and bone or pelvic pain.

Many health benefits have been attributed to the sulfur compounds in garlic, including protection from prostate cancer. Whole garlic extracts were shown to inhibit the growth and multiplication of prostate cancer cell lines by 80 to 90 percent after three days of exposure.[79] Men consuming garlic decreased their risk of developing prostate cancer,[80] and garlic was found to be more effective than onions, which also contain many sulfur compounds. Perhaps the increased efficacy of garlic over onions is due to the garlic-derived compound S-allylmercaptocysteine. Prostate cancer cell lines exposed to S-allylmercaptocysteine experienced growth inhibition and reduced viability.[81] Garlic has the potential to destroy prostate cancer cells. It can therefore be used to reduce the risk of developing prostate cancer and may be beneficial to limit the growth and spread of this disease in the early stages. In more advanced stages, it can be used in combination with doctor-prescribed therapy.

35. RHEUMAToiD ARTHRITIS

Rheumatoid arthritis is an autoimmune disorder in which the immune system mistakenly attacks its own body tissues. The lining of the joints become painfully swollen and can lead to bone erosion and joint deformity over time. Symptoms can spread to other non-joint tissues of the body. It's not known what causes this disease, but genetics combined with environmental triggers are suspected. This chronic disease is without a cure and is managed mostly through medications. Nonsteroidal anti-inflammatory drugs, steroids, or disease-modifying antirheumatic drugs can be prescribed to reduce pain, swelling, and joint damage. Possible side effects include digestive problems, liver and kidney damage, heart problems, thinning of bones, diabetes, weight gain, and severe lung infections.

Garlic has anti-inflammatory properties that can relieve swelling and pain in the joints affected by rheumatoid arthritis. A Russian study supplemented fifteen rheumatoid arthritis patients with a garlic preparation for four to six weeks. A similar control group received conventional antirheumatic therapy. At the end of the trial, 86.5 percent of those consuming the garlic tablets noted improvements in some of their symptoms. The control group did not fare as well.[82]

Garlic also has antioxidant activity and can reduce oxidative stress and injury caused by free radicals in the joints. Methotrexate is a drug used to treat the symptoms of rheumatoid arthritis, but it can damage the kidneys. Seven days of garlic treatment in rats injected with methotrexate found that the antioxidant activity of garlic protected the kidneys and prevented changes in kidney structure.[83] Garlic can be used alone to reduce the symptoms of rheumatoid arthritis or in combination with conventional drug therapy to weaken the negative side effects.

36. RINGWORM

Worms do not actually cause this condition. Ringworm is a fungal infection of the outer layers of skin that is characterized by a red rash that forms a circle, or ring, on the surface of the skin with a clearer patch of skin in the middle. The fungus can affect any area of the body with one or many rings. It is contagious. Even touching bedding, towels, or surfaces that were in contact with the fungus can cause it to adhere to the skin and begin to multiply. Children are most susceptible. Initially, the rash is red, itchy, and flat. If it progresses, the skin can become inflamed with pus-filled blisters. Over-the-counter fungal creams can be used to get rid of the infection, but in severe cases, prescription antifungal medications may be needed.

The safety and potency of garlic's antifungal compound, ajoene, was compared to terbinafine, a common medication used to treat fungal infections of the skin. Sixty men diagnosed with jock itch or athlete's foot were randomized to receive either ajoene gel or ter-binafine cream. After sixty days, the ajoene gel eliminated all signs and symptoms of the fungal infection in 73 percent of the men, while the terbinafine cream was 71 percent effective.[84]

Garlic is a natural herb that can be used to topically treat ring-worm, alleviating not only the intolerable itch but the fungus itself. As a solution, heat freshly cut garlic gently in olive oil for ten min-utes and spread over the infected area when the oil is cool. This can be done several times a day until the infection clears. One batch of garlic oil can be prepared and used each day as long as care is taken to ensure the oil hasn't been contaminated with the fungus.

37. SALMONELLA POISONING

This is a type of food poisoning caused by the *Salmonella* bacteria, which enters the system through contaminated food. This contam-ination can happen to poultry, beef, milk, eggs, and even vegetables during food processing and handling. *Salmonella* is also found in some pets, ducklings, reptiles, hamsters, and other small rodents. Hand-washing is recommended after handling these animals to prevent infection. If *Salmonella* poisoning does happen, it usually occurs within twelve to seventy-two hours after it enters the body. Diarrhea, stomach cramps, and fever develop and can last up to a week. They eventually subside without medication.

There is no way to know if produce contains the *Salmonella* bac-teria because the food looks and smells normal. The best way to

HEALTH

avoid infection is by prevention, so be sure to wash all produce before consuming.

If poisoning does occur, try consuming garlic. Garlic is an anti-bacterial that has been shown to effectively destroy *Salmonella* by interfering with DNA and RNA synthesis.[85] This prevents replication and stops the spread of the infection. Garlic powder is also effective at destroying *Salmonella*, so garlic capsule supplements may be used in place of fresh garlic if appetite is severely depressed.

Some forms of food have the potential to grow bacteria during the manufacturing or processing stages. Chouriço de vinho, a dry pork sausage, is one such food. As it is being made, bacteria can invade the meat and grow, spoiling the product and endangering the consumer. Fresh garlic juice and garlic powder added to both the marinade and the probiotic starter culture was able to control *Salmonella* numbers in the broth during the processing phase. It is recommended that garlic be included in the marinade to ensure the safety of the end product.[86]

Therefore, garlic can be used as a flavorful ingredient in food preparation with the added bonus of bacterial control. It can also be consumed in cases of *Salmonella* poisoning to end the infection sooner.

WELLNESS

PESTS

38. SCLERODERMA

Scleroderma is a chronic disease of the connective tissues, affecting about 300,000 Americans. It is more common in women than men and is usually diagnosed between the ages of twenty-five and fifty-five, although children can develop it too. Scleroderma results

OTHER

from an overproduction of collagen, a fibrous protein that gives tissue strength and elasticity. The body's immune system plays a role in this abnormal collagen production, and research has shown there is a susceptibility gene that raises the probability of getting the disease—but it does not cause it. There are two types: localized scleroderma and systemic scleroderma. The first is relatively mild and affects a few places on the skin or muscles, causing waxy patches of thickened skin. It rarely spreads. The second is more comprehensive and affects connective tissue in many parts of the body, including important internal organs. These organs can become hard and fibrous, causing them to lose function. Problems with the skin have been known to improve over time, but damage to the internal organs tends to worsen. There is no cure for scleroderma, but medications may be taken to dilate blood vessels, prevent the symptoms of acid reflux, relieve pain, or suppress the immune system. Physical therapy can help improve strength and mobility.

A disease with no cure must be continuously managed to ensure the best quality of life possible. Medication takes a toll on the body, and many new symptoms can develop. Using a natural product like garlic as an add-on therapy could help improve symptoms and may even reduce the frequency or dosage needed for medications.

Garlic is classified in traditional European naturopathy as a "heating agent" and is used to increase circulation. Studies do show that garlic has an influence on the functioning of blood vessels. This is important in scleroderma because impaired blood circulation is one of the symptoms that systemic patients suffer. In particular, blood flow to the peripheral blood vessels, like the fingers and toes, is weakened.

HEALTH

WELLNESS

PESTS

OTHER

Standard treatments are often insufficient to improve the situation, but one study gives hope for an answer. In the study, 900 milligrams of dried garlic powder or placebo were given to female sclerosis patients over seven days in conjunction with their current therapies. Garlic significantly reduced platelets from clumping together and lowered red blood cell aggregation. Blood flow was improved, and immediate effects on skin temperature in the peripheral regions were noted.[87] It would be worthwhile for scleroderma patients experiencing cold fingers and toes to make garlic a daily part of their diet.

39. STAPH INFECTION

There are over thirty types of bacterial *Staphylococcus* (staph) infections, but most are caused by *Staphylococcus aureus* (*S. aureus*). These bacteria are responsible for skin infections, pneumonia, food poisoning, blood poisoning, and toxic shock syndrome. Staph skin infections are most common and are usually minor. They look like pimples, blisters, or boils. More severe infections, however, can show red, swollen rashes with pus or drainage. Many people carry these bacteria on their skin or in their noses without any symptoms. The bacteria get into the skin through cuts or scrapes, so it is important to keep wounds clean and to wash hands regularly. If the bacteria invade the body and get into the bloodstream, infections can turn up in numerous organs and become life threatening. Treatment for minor staph infections is usually a course of antibiotics or drainage of infected areas. Severe infections require hospitalization. Many varieties of staph have become resistant to antibiotics. New treatments are needed to continue to fight these ubiquitous bacteria.

The antibacterial activity of whole garlic powder inhibits the growth of *S. aureus*,[88] as does the singular garlic compound ajoene.[89] When preparing food, especially if it contains meat or dairy, consider adding garlic if it pairs well with the other flavors. The garlic will protect the consumer from becoming ill by stopping *Staphylococcus* from multiplying and reaching dangerous levels. Garlic added to samples of hamburger meat that were either refrigerated or frozen had significant inhibition of *Staphylococcus* growth.[90] Garlic can be used to increase the shelf life of hamburgers and reduce the risk of staph infections.

40. THRUSH

When the yeast *C. albicans* overgrows in the lining of the mouth, white lesions develop on the tongue and inner cheeks and may cause redness and soreness. This is called thrush. While *Candida* are normally present in the body, their numbers are kept in check by the immune system. Sometimes when the immune system is weakened by disease or drugs, *Candida* grows out of control and causes an infection. It is most common in babies and the elderly but is also seen in adults with compromised immune systems. This condition is not generally serious, but if left unchecked, the yeast can spread to other areas of the body like the lungs, heart, liver, and digestive tract. Most cases are controlled with antifungal medications.

Garlic is an inexpensive and easily accessible agent that can be used to reduce *Candida* counts and remedy oral thrush. Garlic paste was topically applied to the mouths of fifty-six patients with oral thrush for a period of fourteen days. Clinical signs of redness and pain were reduced. The strength of garlic was comparable to oral clotrimazole, an antifungal medication used to treat yeast infections of the mouth and throat.[91]

Garlic supplements can be taken, or fresh garlic can be cut and put in the mouth for a few minutes before being swallowed. Some may find this too hot, especially children, so it may be more helpful to simmer garlic in water for ten minutes then strain the garlic out and add honey. When the temperature is comfortable, hold each sip of liquid in the mouth for a few seconds before swallowing.

41. TUBERCULOSIS

Tuberculosis is an infectious disease caused by the *Mycobacterium tuberculosis* bacteria. It is spread when an infected person releases bacteria-containing microscopic droplets into the air through coughing, sneezing, laughing, spitting, or talking. If these droplets are inhaled, the bacteria find a new host.

As many as thirteen million people in the United States have the tuberculosis bacteria in its latent form. This means it is present in the body but is in an inactive state and no symptoms are evident. This form is not contagious, but it can turn into active tuberculosis, so treatment is still necessary.

Active tuberculosis is contagious because the bacteria have engaged in multiplying and affect the lungs and sometimes other parts of the body. Symptoms of chronic coughing with or without blood, chest pain, fever, fatigue, and night sweats become evident. Tuberculosis is the top infectious killer worldwide and the leading cause of death in HIV-positive people. Current treatment with antibiotics lasts six to nine months unless the strain is drug resistant, in which case a combination of antibiotics is prescribed for up to thirty months. Many strains of tuberculosis bacteria are resistant to one or more of these drugs, and the fear of more bacteria attaining this ability makes the future of tuberculosis treatment uncertain.

Garlic has been explored as an anti-tuberculosis agent and has shown antibacterial activity against *Mycobacterium tuberculosis* bacteria.[92] One of the compounds in garlic responsible for this activity is allicin. Human white blood cells treated with allicin suppressed activity of the tuberculosis bacteria.[93] In a human model, this means chronic inflammation in the lungs would be diminished or absent. Even drug-resistant strains are susceptible to garlic. Fifteen of them were tested in the presence of garlic, and all activity was inhibited.[94] Garlic should be included in the treatment plans of those with both latent and active tuberculosis, particularly when drug-resistant varieties are present.

42. ULCERATIVE COLITIS

Ulcerative colitis is an inflammatory bowel disease that causes long-lasting inflammation in the innermost lining of the large intestine. The symptoms can vary depending on where the inflammation is located in the large intestine and are usually mild to moderate with periods of remission. Some signs of ulcerative colitis are diarrhea with blood or pus, rectal bleeding, abdominal or rectal pain, an urgency or inability to defecate, fever, fatigue, and weight loss. Treatment options include anti-inflammatory drugs or immunosuppressants. Severe cases may need surgery to remove the colon and rectum.

The anti-inflammatory activity of garlic may be useful in decreasing inflammation of the bowel in ulcerative colitis patients. In rats with ulcerative colitis, garlic oil was administered daily for seven days. Both visible and microscopic changes in the colon were mitigated, decreasing symptoms.[95] Similar findings using alliin from garlic in mice with ulcerative colitis further support this herb in the treatment of this condition. Alliin significantly inhibited weight loss in the mice and decreased the amount of inflammatory cells in the colon.[96] Consuming garlic on a daily basis should help reduce inflammation in the colon and bring relief.

43. VAGINAL TRICHoMONIASIS

Trichomoniasis, also known as trich, is a common sexually transmitted disease caused by the parasite *Trichomonas vaginalis*. About 3.7 million people in the United States have trich, but only about 30 percent know they have it. Most cases go unnoticed because they are asymptomatic.

If symptoms do arise, women can expect a foul-smelling vaginal discharge accompanied by genital itching, painful intercourse, and burning urination. Men may experience itching inside the penis, penile discharge, or a burning sensation during urination or ejaculation. Genital contact with an infected person is needed for contraction of the parasite, and the incubation period is between five and twenty-eight days. Both partners require treatment with antibiotics followed by abstinence from sexual activity until the infection is gone, usually about a week.

The gold standard of treatment for trich is metronidazole, a medication used to treat infections by parasites. The FDA strictly warns that this drug may be hazardous, as its been shown to be carcinogenic in rats and mice. It may also cause serious conditions that affect the nervous system and should only be used when absolutely necessary. Consequently, there is much interest in finding alternative therapies to treat trich.

Garlic shows promise as a phytotherapeutic agent for this. Garlic's effect on *Trichomonas vaginalis* multiplication and motility was examined when exposed to varying concentrations of garlic powder. Garlic completely inhibited both the multiplication and motility of the parasite after twenty-four hours with the highest dose and after ninety-six hours with the lowest dose. These results were comparable to metronidazole, although a larger dose of garlic was needed to obtain the same results.[97] Garlic is safe to consume, with mild side effects, if any. Therefore it can be considered in trich cases to reduce the reliance on metronidazole.

44. VAGINAL YEAST INFECTIONS

Vaginal yeast infections are caused most often by the *Candida albicans* fungus. It is very common, affecting up to 75 percent of women at some point in their lives. This fungus normally lives in the vagina in small numbers, but sometimes, when conditions change to affect the balance of microorganisms, *Candida* grows in numbers, creating an infection. Imbalances can be created from antibiotics, hormonal changes, pregnancy, diabetes, a weakened immune system, too much sugary food in the diet, and stress. Once established, this infection can cause abnormal vaginal discharge, inflammation of vaginal tissue, painful urination, itching, and burning. Over-the-counter antifungal medications can clear the infection within two weeks. These infections have a high reoccurrency rate, and medications will need to be taken each time.

These infections are often treated with fluconazole, an antifungal medication. Some serious side effects to be warned of are liver failure, seizures, and irregular heart rhythm. Garlic, on the other hand, has mild side effects, if any, and has shown to be effective in eliminating a number of *Candida* species. Over a period of seven days, garlic was compared to fluconazole in the treatment of diagnosed cases of vaginal yeast infections. Symptoms improved in 60 percent of the garlic group of patients compared to 71 percent in the fluconazole group. Clinical evaluation of vaginal discharge cultures showed significant improvement in both groups compared to cultures taken before treatment.[98] Garlic can be considered as a safe and effective method to treat vaginal yeast infections and can be consumed daily to prevent infections from reoccurring.

CHAPTER 2

··

ENLIVEN YOUR WELLNESS

··

45. AGING

The process of getting older involves many changes in the body. Arteries stiffen, bones lose density, memory declines, skin thins, and wrinkles appear. The rate at which these processes take place varies from person to person. Genetics and illness play a role in when and how we age, but our diet and lifestyle significantly impact the process. There are many theories of aging, but the free-radical theory is growing in popularity as an explanation. It is thought that free radicals are responsible for age-related damage of cells and tissues. Free radicals are unstable molecules actively looking for an electron. They attack the nearest stable molecule and steal one of their electrons, making that molecule a free radical as well. This begins a chain reaction of creating free radicals that ultimately can destroy the cell.

The key to stopping these free radicals lies in the presence of antioxidants. Because garlic and its components have antioxidant properties, it has been studied in reducing the skin-aging effects of UV exposure. Garlic supplemented in the diet of UV-irradiated mice reduced wrinkle formation, epidermal thickness, and the generation of free radicals. Antioxidant enzymes were increased. Dermal collagen and elastic fiber degradation was suppressed,[99] leaving skin in its firm and elastic condition. It appears that aged garlic is more effective than raw or cooked garlic because it contains higher amounts of organosulfur antioxidants.[100] Daily consumption of garlic may be effective in reducing skin aging induced by UV radiation.

46. ANGINA

Angina is the term for chest pain or discomfort that is a symptom of coronary heart disease. It occurs when there is not enough oxygen-rich blood flowing to the heart due to the narrowing or blockage of one or more arteries leading to the heart. There are two types. The first, stable angina, is usually triggered by physical exercise and lasts a short time. It feels like pressure or squeezing in the chest, and the discomfort may extend to the neck, jaw, shoulder, back, or arms. Women may experience different symptoms like nausea, shortness of breath, extreme fatigue, and abdominal pain. The second type, unstable angina, is more severe and can cause chest pain at any time, even at rest. It tends to last longer and is usually caused by a blood clot that partially or totally blocks blood flow to the heart. The result can be a heart attack. Mild stable angina usually just requires adopting a healthier lifestyle. Medications like statins, beta blockers, calcium channel blockers, nitroglycerin, aspirin, and other blood clotting drugs can help improve blood flow. Unstable angina may need an angioplasty and stenting or coronary bypass surgery to remove any blockages and restore blood flow to the heart.

Among garlic's many benefits is its antithrombotic activity. It has the ability to decrease blood clot formation by preventing blood platelets from sticking together. This was demonstrated in patients with unstable angina who received intravenous garlic injections for ten days. Symptoms improved by 82 percent, and clinical evaluation by electrocardiogram saw a 62 percent correction in blood flow.[101] Garlic can be used as a daily prophylactic therapy to prevent angina or decrease the incidence or severity of angina episodes.

47. BLOOD THINNER

Blood clots are necessary to stop bleeding, but they can also form in places in the body where they can be dangerous. In the arteries and veins, blood clots can form in an attempt to repair tissue damage by laying down layers of fibrin and platelets. This is a problem because these clots slow the flow of blood. They can block blood vessels completely at their site of origin, or they can break off and plug a vein or artery elsewhere in the body. This can be extremely serious and lead to heart attack or stroke. Depending on where the clot is located, treatment can be with either anticoagulation medications or with acetaminophen or ibuprofen to manage pain and inflammation. Some side effects of anticoagulants include severe bruising, bleeding gums, vomiting blood, chest pain, and prolonged nosebleeds.

Garlic's ability to inhibit platelet aggregation as well as reduce LDL cholesterol and blood pressure make it an excellent choice to improve blood flow and decrease the incidence of blood clots. Garlic's efficacy was demonstrated in subjects with normal lipid profiles who ingested aged garlic extract each day for thirteen weeks. Blood was drawn from these subjects at the end of the test period and treated with ADP, a compound naturally occurring in the body that causes blood platelets to stick together, forming clots. The blood of garlic-ingesting subjects showed significantly inhibited platelet aggregation.[102] Garlic is just as effective in those with coronary artery disease, who often show high levels of lipids, like cholesterol. Daily garlic administration significantly increased the breakdown of clots in addition to reducing serum cholesterol.[103] Those at risk of cardiovascular disease or cerebrovascular accidents may want to consider consuming garlic on a daily basis as a preventative measure.

48. CAVITIES

The mouth is full of bacteria. Some are helpful, and others are harmful. The harmful bacteria form a sticky, colorless substance called plaque that adheres to the teeth and gum line. Plaque loves to feed on sugars and starches, so nearly every meal provides plaque with fuel for growth. As the bacteria in the plaque feed on the sugars, they produce acids. These acids demineralize the tooth surface by extracting calcium and phosphate from the enamel. Saliva tries to neutralize the acids and provide the missing minerals so that the teeth enamel can remineralize. When demineralization happens faster than remineralization, the tooth begins to decay, creating holes called cavities. Cavities are a major oral health concern and affect up to 90 percent of schoolchildren and the majority of adults. The only treatment for cavities is to drill out the decay and fill the hole with composite resins, porcelain, or amalgams.

Once a cavity has begun, the process cannot be reversed. The best course of action is to prevent tooth decay before it starts. A good oral hygiene routine is essential and should involve flossing once a day and brushing twice a day. Reducing sugar consumption can also help to lower acid output from the bacteria that cause enamel erosion.

HEALTH

WELLNESS

PESTS

OTHER

There are a number of commercially available mouth rinses that contain ingredients that can get rid of the bacteria, but the side effects can include vomiting, diarrhea, tooth staining, and a disturbance of oral and intestinal flora. Natural plants, like garlic, can be effective at preventing tooth decay with far fewer side effects. Garlic with lime was compared to chlorhexidine (antiseptic), sodium fluoride (remineralization), fluoride with essential oils (remineralization and antiseptic), and alum (antiseptic) for their abilities to destroy cavity-causing bacteria. After chlorhexidine, garlic with lime was found to be the most effective mouth rinse to destroy unwanted bacteria and protect the teeth from decay.[104] Garlic is even effective on multidrug-resistant strains of *Streptococcus mutans* that contribute to cavities. In ninety-two isolates of this bacteria from carious teeth, 30 percent were resistant to four or more antibiotics. None of them were resistant to garlic.[105] Using garlic as an ingredient in mouthwashes or toothpastes could help reduce the incidence of cavities.

49. CHRONIC FATIGUE SYNDROME

This syndrome is characterized by extreme fatigue that is not relieved by rest. It is accompanied by headaches, muscle pain, joint pain, sleep problems, tender lymph nodes, or memory loss. It is not known what causes chronic fatigue, but hormonal imbalances, some viral infections, or impaired immune systems may be triggers. Restrictions in daily activity are common, and those with chronic fatigue often feel depressed. To aid with the symptoms, antidepressants are frequently taken to help with mood, pain, and sleep.

Garlic has broad-spectrum antimicrobial activity and can protect the body from a wide range of infections that drain the body of energy. Patients with chronic fatigue syndrome (CFS) suffer from abnormally depressed immune-system functions. This may be attributed in part to the presence of chronic intestinal candidiasis. Eighty-three percent of CFS patients that underwent an anti-*Candida* protocol to treat yeast infections achieved a reduction in their CFS symptoms, suggesting a strong correlation between CFS and candidiasis.[106] Garlic has been shown to effectively destroy *Candida albicans*, the fungus causing candidiasis. It causes oxidative stress to several tested species of *Candida* and damages the cells, causing death.[107] If you are diagnosed with CFS, consuming garlic on a daily basis may remove the fungus responsible for compromising the immune system, allowing for improved function and a return of energy.

50. COGNITIVE FUNCTION

The attainment and processing of knowledge is a direct function of cognitive or mental processes that include perception, memory, reasoning, judgment, attention, and language. Each person is unique and will differ in how they see and react to the world around them. Genetics accounts for the majority of cognitive variation seen in the general population. Environmental factors and physiological processes make up the rest. Chemical imbalances and changes in metabolic pathways can bring a noticeable change in cognition over time. Some of these processes can be triggered with age, dietary deficiencies, or exogenous chemical or pathogen exposure, leading to the impairment of memory and thinking skills.

Memory loss and difficulty learning new tasks are common in some forms of amnesia. Amnesic mice supplemented with garlic for three weeks saw a partial reversal of amnesia in the short term and a significant improvement in learning over the long term.[108] Another condition affecting cognition is oxidative stress resulting from insulin resistance. Obese rats with this condition had cognitive deficits which were improved after four weeks of garlic treatment.[109] Even lead-induced memory problems can be ameliorated with garlic. It lowered the lead content in the brain tissues of rats and protected against oxidative damage. The effect was comparable to the protection provided by vitamin C, commonly used to overcome lead toxicity.[110]

51. COLDS

Common colds are respiratory illnesses caused by viruses. They are highly contagious, and a person can become infected by touching a surface such as a doorknob, stair railing, or bathroom faucet. If the virus gets on the hands and the person then touches their mouth or nose, the virus nestles into the mucosal lining there. Another surefire way of getting the virus into the system is breathing in air near someone who is coughing or sneezing due to a cold.

There are many different viruses that cause colds. Unless the body has fought the exact virus before, it won't have the right antibodies ready to fight it when it enters the body. The immune system begins an attack against the new virus, and the dreaded symptoms set in. A sore throat, a runny or stuffed nose, sneezing, and a cough are the hallmarks of a cold. There is no shortage of over-the-counter cold medications, and they are available for every possible symptom. Take a walk down the pharmacy aisle to see antihistamines, decongestants, nasal sprays, cough suppressants, and throat lozenges.

The rhinovirus is the most common infectious viral agent in humans and the main cause of the common cold. Fresh garlic extract destroys this virus, possibly through inhibiting its absorption into host cells.[111] Garlic also boosts the immune system to provide better protection against invading viruses. Healthy subjects recruited to test the effects of garlic on the immune system as well as cold and flu symptoms found that those consuming aged garlic extract had higher numbers of important immune cells. These specific cells attack and destroy host cells that have been infected with viruses. In addition, the group consuming garlic had fewer colds. Their colds lasted a shorter amount of time, and symptoms were less severe.[112] When an allicin-containing garlic supplement was studied, participants were afflicted with significantly fewer colds over the treatment period between November and February compared to those who did not take garlic.[113] An inexpensive and effective home remedy to combat these symptoms is to include garlic in the diet.

52. CORNS

A localized, hardened bump of skin surrounded by softer inflamed skin that is painful when pressed or touched is a corn. They typically occur on the tops and sides of the toes or even between them.

HEALTH

WELLNESS

PESTS

OTHER

They arise from bone pressure or friction against the skin. The first step to removing painful and unsightly corns is to remove the source of pressure. This may mean switching to shoes that fit properly. Shoes that are too loose may cause friction from repeated sliding, and shoes that are too tight may compress the foot, adding prolonged pressure. Wear socks to reduce friction and consider donut-shaped adhesive pads that surround the corn, taking pressure off the area. Bandages medicated with salicylic acid to soften the dead skin are also available, but this can damage healthy skin too. If no underlying health problems exist, corns can be gradually removed at home. Soak the skin in warm water until the corn softens, then gently remove the top layers of skin that easily flake off. Be careful not to take off too much skin; this will be painful and expose cracks or tears in the skin that can open the corn to infection.

A gentle way to remove corns is to apply garlic directly to the area. When the skin forms corns, the body responds by sending the protein fibrin to the area to begin wound healing. The fibrin molecules are like long threads that interlace and form a mesh over the corn. Garlic disintegrates this fibrin tissue and separates the corn from the skin.[114]

To remove a corn, cut a slice of a garlic clove and rub it over the corn so that the juice covers the area. Then secure the garlic to the corn with a bandage. It is more convenient to do this at bedtime. In the morning, discard the garlic and wash the foot. Repeat each night. After about a week, the corn should be gone. This, of course, depends on the size of the corn. Larger corns with more hardened tissue will take longer.

53. COUGHS

Coughing is the body's reaction to irritated airways or a reflex action to remove mucus and foreign material from the lungs and upper airways. Smoke, dust, allergies, asthma, some medicines, bronchospasms, or an inhaled object can cause dry coughs. Wet coughs result when mucus drains down the back of the throat from the sinuses or comes up the airways from the lungs. Infections, viruses, lung disease, postnasal drip, and smoking can cause mucus-induced wet coughs. People commonly buy expectorant medications to break up congestion and suppressants to try to stop the cough. These medications can become addictive and cause dizziness, drowsiness, nausea, and vomiting, even at recommended dosages.

Research shows that garlic is commonly used for the relief of coughs in complementary alternative medicine.[115] Garlic has been proven to reduce the incidence and severity of cold symptoms, wet cough being one of them. It works indirectly by boosting the immune system to rid the body of cold-producing viruses and directly by inactivating the viruses themselves. With the source of infection defeated, the body stops producing mucus and the need to cough subsides. The next time a cough disrupts your day or keeps you up all night, try taking garlic cough syrup.

GARLIC COUGH SYRUP

3 cloves crushed garlic
1 cup filtered water
1/4 cup raw honey

1. Simmer the crushed garlic in water for twenty minutes. Remove from heat and strain out the garlic.
2. Stir in the honey until it is well incorporated. Take 1 teaspoon as needed. Store the syrup in a glass jar in the pantry.

54. DANDRUFF

Dandruff is a chronic condition marked by the flaking of skin cells on the scalp. The flakes are visible as white, oily-looking specks of skin on the hair and shoulders. It is not a dangerous condition, but it can be embarrassing for some people. One of the leading causes of dandruff is a condition known as seborrheic dermatitis. It is thought to develop when *Malassezia* fungi, commonly found on the oil glands of the skin, promote the development of flaky white or yellow scales on the scalp. Skin in these areas shed as dandruff. Mild cases are easy to treat with daily cleansing to reduce oil and skin cell buildup. Other cases are more difficult and may need medicated shampoos. Some shampoos contain antifungal agents to kill the microbes. Others work by slowing the death rate of skin cells to reduce buildup and flaking.

Garlic is praised as an excellent home remedy for dandruff caused by seborrheic dermatitis and boosts the body's immune system to help fight *Malassezia* infections. It was shown to dose-dependently inhibit the growth of ninety strains of various fungi, including *Malassezia* strains.[116] This points to garlic as a promising candidate to control *Malassezia* numbers in the oil secretions of the scalp and prevent the development of seborrheic dermatitis and the resulting dandruff.

To treat dandruff, garlic can be crushed and added to olive oil. After infusion for twenty minutes or more, this mixture can be rubbed into the scalp and left in place for 15 minutes. Rinse and shampoo as normal.

55. DENTURE-INDUCED STOMATITIS

Gum disease, tooth decay, or injury can all damage teeth to the point where they fall out or need to be removed. Dentures can replace missing teeth, thus improving facial appearance and the ability to eat and speak. Complete dentures replace all the teeth in the mouth, and partial dentures replace only the teeth that are missing. Dentures should be removed at night and cleaned with a soft-bristle toothbrush to remove food, plaque, bacteria, and yeast. Storing the dentures overnight in a glass of water will prevent the dentures from drying out and warping. If they are not cleaned properly, dentures can cause irritation of the gums and bad breath.

Brushing dentures does remove food and plaque but is not very effective in removing bacteria and yeasts. If a disinfecting agent is not used in addition to brushing, the denture wearer runs the risk of infection of the mucosal membranes in the mouth. This is often caused by *Candida*, yeast commonly found in the mouth. If left alone, they multiply and thrive on the gums underneath the dentures. This causes a condition known as denture-induced stomatitis, which is inflammation and redness of the gums.

Nystatin is an antifungal drug commonly used to treat denture stomatitis. It has a bitter taste and can cause mouth irritation, nausea, diarrhea, or upset stomach. This drug was compared to garlic for the elimination of *Candida* infections in the mouths of patients who were diagnosed with denture stomatitis. Over a four-week period, patients in both groups had significant reduction in the extent of their infections, but those taking garlic were more satisfied with their treatment.[117] This may have been due to garlic's lack of side effects and more pleasing taste.

Garlic shows superiority to other antifungal medications, like fluconazole. This is especially important because some fungal species are resistant to fluconazole. A number of *Candida* species were isolated from the dentures of patients and exposed to either garlic essential oil or fluconazole. All species were destroyed by garlic, but a small percentage of them were resistant to fluconazole and continued to thrive. In further investigations, *Candida* cells that clump together to form biofilms—a slimy film of yeast cells that adheres to dentures—were very resistant to destruction by fluconazole. Garlic, however, proved to be more potent and eliminated the majority of *Candida* cells.[118] Using garlic in combination with or in place of the antifungal drugs may clear up infections more quickly and in a safer, gentler way for the body.

56. DIARRHEA

Diarrhea describes loose, watery stools. It is very common and usually lasts a few days, although prolonged diarrhea can indicate a medical condition like irritable bowel syndrome. Stomach cramps and pain, bloating, fever, nausea, and vomiting often accompany diarrhea. It occurs when the stool moves too quickly through the colon so that the colon doesn't have time to absorb enough liquid from it. The main culprits in causing diarrhea are viruses, bacteria, and parasites. Food intolerance and many medications can also cause diarrhea in susceptible people. If diarrhea persists for more than a few days, doctors may prescribe antibiotics if the cause is bacterial or parasitic.

Some pathogenic organisms known to cause diarrhea in humans (*E. coli*, *Salmonella*, *Shigella*, and *Proteus mirabilis*) were exposed to raw garlic extract and the broad-spectrum antibiotic drugs ciprofloxacin and ampicillin. Garlic was superior to ampicillin in its effectiveness on all four types of bacteria and was similar to ciprofloxacin in its exceptional antimicrobial activity. Ampicillin has been prescribed indiscriminately for many years, and strains of bacteria are becoming resistant to it, decreasing its efficacy. This type of resistance is not known to occur in garlic.[119] Garlic can be consumed in cases of diarrhea to destroy the infectious bacteria and resolve all symptoms.

57. DIURETIC

Sometimes called water pills, diuretics are drugs or other substances that force the kidneys to remove excess water and salt from the blood and tissues. The excess is excreted through the urine. Diuretics are often prescribed when medical conditions cause a buildup of excess fluid in tissues. This creates pressure and can lead to a number of dangerous health conditions. By removing water, pressure is reduced in the tissues and makes processes like breathing and pumping blood easier. As such, diuretics are often used to

HEALTH

WELLNESS

PESTS

OTHER

reduce blood volume in those with high blood pressure, preserving the structural integrity of the arteries and reducing the risk for heart attack and stroke.

Garlic is a natural diuretic that can be used in place of prescribed diuretic pills in mild forms of high blood pressure or when the body is feeling bloated. Remember that garlic taken with other diuretics may induce the loss of too much water, resulting in dehydration. If taking prescription diuretics, always consult a doctor before supplementing with garlic. You can expect the response to reach its maximum effect thirty to forty minutes after ingesting garlic, with the kidneys returning to normal function after 100 to 150 minutes—that is, if we were dogs. Human reaction time will be different, but we can use the dog model as a general guideline. In a study on the use of garlic as a diuretic, the dogs not only had an increase in fluid output but a simultaneous decrease in arterial blood pressure.[120] Taking this natural herb is definitely a safe and effective way to rid the body of too much fluid in humans. Caution is advised in feeding garlic to dogs, however. It contains thiosulfate, which is toxic to dogs and can cause digestive distress and anemia.

58. ENLARGED PROSTATE

As men age, their prostate gland gets larger and pinches the urethra. This narrows the tube through which urine flows from the bladder through the penis to the outside of the body. This can lead to urinary retention, frequent urination, a weak urine stream, or a delayed start to the urine stream. Less than half of men with enlarged prostates actually experience symptoms, but if they are bothersome, decrease liquid intake and avoid diuretics. Stay away from medications that contain decongestants or antihistamines because they contain ingredients that can increase symptoms. In more severe cases, medications can be taken to relax the muscles of the bladder and prostate to allow easier urine flow or reduce the size of the prostate gland. Surgical removal of the prostate is possible, if needed.

A large case study in men, with and without enlarged prostates, investigated the relationship between the dietary intake of garlic and onions (which share some of the same bioactive sulfur compounds) and the prevalence of enlarged prostates. Interestingly, it was found that the more garlic and onions consumed in the diet, the lower the chance of having an enlarged prostate.[121] Garlic suppresses the cellular growth of the gland and decreases inflammation of the tissue.[122] Both these processes inhibit the prostate from becoming bigger and affecting bladder function.

59. EXERCISE-INDUCED MUSCLE SORENESS

After months of inactivity, going out for a competitive game of flag football or a vigorous evening run with a friend may seem like a good idea. However, the discomfort of trying to move about the next day when every muscle is stiff and sore will squelch that belief. You might want to take preventative measures to guard against injury-induced muscle pain or aches from overuse before the next time.

Muscle aches can also result from tension, stress, or disease. The pain can be anywhere in the body and last from several hours to months. If exercise induced, muscle pain results from microscopic tears in the muscle fibers, while if disease related, it can be caused by inflammation.

To get ready for an intense bout of exercise, try adding garlic to the diet before the big day and continue for a few days after to reduce muscle soreness. Garlic supplemented to well-trained athletes for fourteen days prior to a downhill treadmill run and for two days after reduced exercise-induced muscle soreness. Those in the garlic group had higher levels of antioxidants, which reduces oxidative stress and, consequently, muscle damage. Significantly lower levels of creatine kinase, a molecule that rises after skeletal muscle damage, and interleukin 6, a protein that promotes inflammation, were measured. Perceived muscle soreness after exercise was also lower as compared to the control group, who also ran on the treadmill but did not supplement with garlic.[123]

60. EXERCISE PERFORMANCE

Aerobic exercise improves fitness by increasing heart and breathing rates for a duration of longer than a few minutes. Blood gets pumped around the body, delivering oxygen to the cells to keep the muscles working. Increasing fitness improves not only physical health but mental and emotional health as well. Regular aerobic exercise strengthens the heart, makes the muscles more efficient at consuming oxygen, and increases the number of mitochondria in the muscle cells. These increase endurance and more efficiently burn fat and carbohydrates. Running, walking, biking, and swimming are some examples of aerobic activity.

It's important to work anaerobically too. This type of exercise is short and intense. It relies on oxygen already stored in the muscles and is primarily performed to build muscle. Lifting weights or resistance training using body weight can do this. Weight training breaks down muscles, and during repair, there is a new and larger growth of muscle tissue. It is theorized that the muscles get larger to protect the body from future stresses.

Many of us have a goal to increase our fitness, and there are numerous products on the market that promise to do this by improving stamina or building muscle. Some of these may work, but they often have a long list of questionable ingredients. Garlic can be used as a potential agent to increase exercise performance without the adverse side effects of some of the other products available. Healthy trained males were divided into groups that received either 900 milligrams of garlic powder or a placebo three hours before a graded treadmill test. After two weeks, the men switched groups and performed the test again, this time with the other test drug (garlic powder or placebo).[124] The results indicate that garlic significantly increases VO_2 max, which is the maximum rate of oxygen consumption measured during incremental exercise that determines the cardiorespiratory fitness of the subject. Those with improved VO_2 max levels tend to increase endurance capacity during prolonged exercise.

61. FEVER

Fever is a temporary increase in the body's temperature. It is not an illness but a sign that something unusual is happening in the body.

Mild fevers should be left untreated to allow the immune system to take care of the cause. Higher fevers are of more concern and require some intervention. Sweating, chills, fatigue, muscle weakness, and headache may accompany fevers. They are generally caused by viruses, bacteria, some medications, sunburn, inflammatory conditions, and malignant tumors. Over-the-counter medications such as aspirin, acetaminophen, or prescribed antibacterial drugs are effective in reducing fever but come with risks. Antibiotics destroy good intestinal bacteria, causing digestive upset; overuse of acetaminophen can cause kidney and liver damage; and aspirin can cause stomach pain, unusual bleeding, and weakness.

Using herbal remedies for body complaints and symptoms is becoming increasingly popular. In sixteen randomly selected healthcare facilities in Trinidad, patients that commonly used herbs in managing their health were selected to provide information on specific usage. They believed so strongly in the potency of these herbs that 87 percent thought they were as effective as doctor-prescribed medication. Over one hundred different herbs were cited, but garlic was the most popular. Of the 265 participants, 48 percent used garlic, mostly to reduce fevers, coughs, and symptoms of the common cold.[125] Despite the absence of clinical trials studying garlic on fever reduction in humans, its validity is supported by widespread and long-standing use. This is further backed by a study in which pigs were infected with a porcine virus. Those fed garlic had lower rectal temperatures than pigs in the control group who were not fed garlic.[126]

62. FLU

Seasonal flu is a respiratory illness caused by influenza A and B viruses. The flu is contagious, and a person can become infected by touching a surface with the virus and transferring it to their mouth or nose. Here, the virus nestles into the mucosal lining and begins to replicate. Contaminated people who cough or sneeze cause the virus to become airborne. Simply breathing in this air can begin an infection.

Symptoms can be mild or severe, and in certain cases, they can be fatal. Symptoms include a fever, sore throat, runny or stuffed nose, cough, fatigue, muscle aches, and headaches. At its onset, antiviral drugs can be taken to shorten the duration of the illness by one or two days and lessen the severity of symptoms.

Each year, many people opt to get a flu vaccine to try to prevent seasonal influenza. This does not guarantee that you won't get sick, however. Those that succumb to the flu may choose to take antiviral drugs, but these have possible side effects that include nausea, vomiting, diarrhea, and headaches. To avoid these, try aged garlic extract instead. One study testing the effect of daily aged garlic consumption versus placebo on the reduction of cold and flu symptoms recruited 120 healthy humans. After forty-five days, immune system cells responsible for killing viruses were more active in garlic users. At the end of the study, participants in the garlic group who contracted flu viruses had fewer and less severe symptoms than those in the control group. They also had fewer absences at work and school.[127] Garlic enhances immune function and enables the body to better ward off viruses.

63. HAY FEVER

Allergic reactions that occur seasonally when certain environmental irritants are more abundant, such as pollen in the spring, can cause irritations that are similar to the symptoms of a cold. They result in a runny nose; itchy, watery eyes; frequent sneezing; sinus congestion; and possibly headaches. It's not just outdoor allergens, though. Indoor allergens like dust mites or pet dander can induce hay fever symptoms at any time of the year.

Hay fever happens when the immune system reacts abnormally to these harmless substances. It sees them as unwelcome invaders and attacks them by producing specific antibodies that identify the allergen as harmful to the body. Every time a person comes in contact with that allergen, the allergic response is activated.

There is no cure for allergies, but there are many over-the-counter and prescription drugs available to help ease symptoms. Among these are antihistamines, decongestants, and corticosteroids. They can cause drowsiness, high blood pressure, insomnia, irritability, restricted urine flow, muscle weakness, fluid retention, and weight gain—and these are just some of the side effects. This seems like trading one set of symptoms for another.

Garlic can help boost the immune system to increase its ability to handle stress, toxins, and irritants. A stronger immune system reduces allergic potential. Aged garlic extract supplemented to healthy human participants increased their immune cell function and reduced the severity of cold symptoms,[128] which share many of the same symptoms as those suffering from hay fever. Garlic also contains apigenin,[129] a flavonoid compound that is a strong anti-inflammatory. Apigenin inhibits specific proteins that are associated with allergies and the allergic response. Consider consuming garlic on a daily basis if allergies are year round. If they are seasonal, start taking garlic a few weeks before allergies begin and continue until the irritant is gone and symptoms have disappeared.

64. HEADACHES AND MIGRAINES

A headache is a pain in any part of the head and may be sharp, dull, or throbbing. It can last from under an hour to several days. Migraines are severe headaches that cause intense pain, usually on one side of the head, and are accompanied by nausea, vomiting, and sensitivity to light and sound. Migraines can come with warning signs such as blind spots in the field of vision, flashes of light, or tingling sensations on the face, arms, or legs. Migraines can be so severe that the person can't function normally and often requires rest and isolation to recover.

Causes of migraines are different for everyone. Some triggers could be changes in hormone levels, food allergies, stress, some medications, sensory stimuli, or changes in the environment, like a fall in barometric pressure from an approaching storm. Regular headaches can be caused by a multitude of factors, from dehydration to too little sleep to infections. They may also be symptoms of disease. Pain-relieving medications are commonly used to deal with the symptoms. In the case of migraines, anti-nausea medications are also prescribed.

Garlic has been suggested for centuries as a headache treatment. Perhaps it is the ability of garlic to thin the blood that can reduce the risk of headaches, but more likely it is a combination of factors that makes it effective. Garlic oil was given to adult rats with induced cortical spreading depression (CSD), which is thought to be an underlying cause of migraine auras and pain. Garlic oil suppressed the severity of CSD, although duration was not affected.[130] This suggests garlic can decrease the intensity of headaches and migraines but not how long they last.

Headaches resulting from chemical exposure, like lead, can also be very painful. Garlic oil was able to significantly reduce headache symptoms in men with high blood lead levels in addition to removing the lead from the blood. It could be argued that the disappearance of the headaches naturally followed the removal of lead from the body, but another substance, d-penicillamine, was also used to remove lead in comparable subjects, and this medication did not alleviate headache symptoms.[131]

A fresh garlic clove can be eaten to provide headache relief, or garlic tea may be more preferable. Another way to try garlic is to inhale the steam from garlic cloves boiled in water. Be careful not to burn the nostrils.

65. HEMORRHoIDS

Hemorrhoids are swollen veins in the rectum and anus. The walls of the veins can stretch and cause the blood vessels to bulge. Internal hemorrhoids are inside the rectum and can bleed into the stool. This area has few pain receptors, so hemorrhoids here generally do not hurt. External hemorrhoids are located on the anus, where there are more pain-sensing nerves. These can be quite sore, especially during a bowel movement. They develop from a buildup of pressure in the lower rectum that can affect the flow of blood and cause the veins to swell. Straining during a bowel movement, pregnancy, or obesity can cause them. Hemorrhoids are extremely common and can explain bleeding, itching, pain, and inflammation. Topical creams or suppositories, cold packs, and oral pain relievers can help subside symptoms.

High blood pressure can put too much pressure on the small veins in the rectum, forming hemorrhoids. Garlic significantly lowers high blood pressure in hypertensive patients[132] and may reduce the risk of developing hemorrhoids. If they are already present, the pain and inflammation can be alleviated by raw garlic because garlic is an anti-inflammatory. As it reduces swelling of the tissue, pain and itching subside.

Insert a peeled clove of garlic coated in coconut oil about an inch into the rectum. Leave it overnight and allow the next day's bowel movement to remove it from the body. Repeat each night until the hemorrhoids shrink and symptoms disappear.

66. KIDNEY PROTECTION

Injury to the kidneys can cause them to lose their ability to remove waste products from the blood and balance fluids. Acute cases of renal failure are when the kidneys suddenly lose their filtering ability and dangerous levels of waste products build up in the blood. This happens over a short period of time and requires intensive treatment. Complete recovery is possible. Chronic renal failure is progressive and irreversible. Symptoms are due to the buildup of waste products in the body and include weakness, shortness of breath, fatigue, and confusion. Abnormal heart rhythms and sudden death can follow. Prevention is the best course of action and involves controlling blood pressure and diabetes. If the disease has progressed too far, dialysis or transplants may be needed.

Acetaminophen is a very popular medication taken to reduce pain and fever. If used habitually, and especially when taken with alcohol, it can cause structural and functional damage to the kidneys. Diallyl disulfide derived from garlic can protect the kidneys from this type of damage. Consuming garlic before acetaminophen administration significantly lowered kidney damage, abnormal structural changes, and the destruction of kidney cells in rats.[133] Next time you reach for acetaminophen, remember to take some garlic beforehand to ensure your kidneys remain safe.

67. LICE

Every year, it seems children are sent home from school with a note warning parents that there is an outbreak of head lice in the school. These tiny insects that infest children's (and adults') scalps are a source of panic and embarrassment, although having lice is not a sign of poor personal hygiene.

Lice feed on the blood of the scalp and are readily transferred from one person to another through direct contact. They can also fall off the head and land on the carpet, bedding, towels, and stuffed animals, where they can lay their eggs and continue to grow for another day or two. A person may be infected for several weeks before itching (an allergic reaction to the louse saliva) begins.

The lice and nits (eggs) are difficult to see, but a close look around the ears and neckline may provide the best chance of glimpsing them. Over-the-counter and prescription medicated shampoos are used to kill the adult lice. The eggs are hard to get rid of because they adhere to the hair shaft with a sticky substance that is difficult to wash out. A second treatment of medicated shampoo is recommended when the nits hatch.

The strong fragrance of garlic is thought to suffocate lice, therefore nymphs and adult lice can be removed from the scalp with a garlic treatment. Adding apple cider vinegar to the formula loosens the nits from the hair shaft so the eggs can be removed as well. Repeat the treatment each night for up to a week until all lice and eggs are gone.

LICE TREATMENT

1 bulb garlic
1 tablespoon apple cider vinegar
2 tablespoons coconut oil

1. Grind all the cloves in the garlic bulb to a paste. Mix with the apple cider vinegar and coconut oil.
2. Apply the mixture to the scalp. Massage in thoroughly and leave for 30 minutes. Rinse and shampoo as normal.

68. LIVER PROTECTION

The liver is the largest internal organ in the body. It filters toxins out of the bloodstream to prevent them from damaging tissues.

HEALTH

WELLNESS

PESTS

OTHER

When the liver tissue itself becomes damaged, it has the ability to regenerate and make new, healthy tissue. When the damage gets too extensive, however, liver disease sets in, and the liver no longer functions as it should. A number of conditions can cause liver disease, including hepatitis A, B, and C; cirrhosis of the liver; nonalcoholic fatty liver disease; and alcoholic hepatitis. Poisons, medications, and viruses are other causes. Symptoms include abdominal swelling and pain, bruising, fatigue, loss of appetite, and jaundice.

The liver is constantly bombarded with hazardous compounds that threaten the health of various tissues in the body or the individual as a whole. If not metabolized into harmless compounds or excreted out of the body, these compounds become toxic to the liver and impair its critical functions. It is imperative that the liver be protected so that it continues to defend the rest of the body.

Acetaminophen is one such medication known to induce liver toxicity. It is one of the most popular painkillers in the United States, with billions of these pills taken each year. When using acetaminophen, make sure to consume garlic with it. When garlic was taken half an hour after acetaminophen, it suppressed acute liver injury and prevented overdose death in mice.[134]

Single-clove garlic can also protect the liver from one of the most potent liver toxins, carbon tetrachloride. The antioxidants in garlic can provide protection against this compound, which, if left unchecked, can cause severe damage to the structural tissues of the liver.[135] Garlic can even work synergistically with other medicines to greatly improve the effectiveness of the drugs. Diphenyl dimethyl bicarboxylate (DDB), used as a medicine in some countries to prevent liver damage in chronic hepatitis patients, works much more effectively when garlic oil is added to it.[136]

69. PREMENSTRUAL DISORDER

Women of childbearing years often experience pain and cramping just before or during the first few days of menstruation. Pain can be mild to severe and is described as a dull, throbbing ache in the lower abdomen, hips, back, and thighs. It usually lasts twelve to seventy-two hours and, for some, can prevent normal activities for several days. It happens when the muscles of the woman's uterus contract too strongly and put pressure on nearby blood vessels. Oxygen to muscle tissue of the uterus is temporarily cut off, and pain results. Primary menstrual cramps usually occur each menstrual cycle and can be associated with other symptoms like nausea, vomiting, diarrhea, and fatigue. They are differentiated from secondary menstrual pain, which has an underlying cause like a reproductive disorder or infection.

The main objective in managing this condition is to reduce pain and treat the symptoms. Over-the-counter pain relievers and hormone birth control are used to relieve pain.

Garlic was also shown to relieve symptoms. Women divided into two groups received either a supplement containing 150 milligrams of garlic and vitamins or a placebo pill twice a day. After six months, the severity of symptoms associated with premenstrual syndrome were reduced, including aching menstrual cramps and breast pain.[137] It would be helpful for women experiencing this monthly syndrome to consume garlic on a daily basis to reduce debilitating symptoms and improve their quality of life.

70. RADIATION PROTECTION

Radiation is energy in particle or wave form that can cause gene mutations from long-term exposure and increase the risk of cancer. Large doses over a short period of time cause radiation sickness and lead to nausea, hair loss, organ failure, or even death. Outside, there is constant exposure to radiation from the UV rays of the sun. Indoors, medical procedures using X-rays and tomography scans emit doses. In the home, some of the culprits are microwaves, wireless internet connections, and mobile phones. Living in the modern world, it is impossible to avoid radiation exposure if one is to interact in society. The best thing to do to minimize the effects of exposure is to take preventative measures, whether it be from the UVA and UVB rays of the sun or from surrounding electronics.

Several sulfur compounds derived from garlic show potential as radioprotective agents. Allylmethylsulfide decreased cell damage from free radicals generated in mice after exposure to X-rays. It also suppressed the activation of disease-promoting enzymes.[138] Sodium 2-propenyl thiosulfate (2PTS) significantly decreased X-ray-induced DNA damage in rat and mice cells when the cells were preincubated in 2PTS for forty-eight hours prior to radiation exposure.[139] Eating garlic on a daily basis could provide protection to the body from environmental radiation exposure. As a precaution, it would also be a good idea to consume some for a few days both before and after any procedures requiring irradiation.

71. SHORTNESS OF BREATH

Having difficulty breathing can be very frightening. A number of triggers like high altitude, obesity, strenuous exercise, or extreme temperatures can cause shortness of breath. In many cases, however, this is a symptom of certain medical conditions, particularly those affecting the heart and lungs. Shortness of breath is often accompanied by low oxygen levels in the blood of the arteries. This can be due to the lungs not absorbing enough oxygen from the air or the blood not transporting enough oxygen to the tissues. Whatever the cause, breathing is affected.

People with hepatopulmonary syndrome have shortness of breath and low oxygen levels in their arterial blood. Garlic has been shown to improve breathing in these patients by improving their blood oxygen levels. Forty percent of subjects administered garlic powder capsules each day for six months increased the amount of oxygen in their blood by at least 10 mmHg or decreased the difference in the amount of oxygen in lung cells compared to arterial cells, meaning more oxygen was being transported throughout the body.[140] In children with this syndrome, garlic powder capsules also increased blood oxygen levels by 10 mmHg, but this time in 53 percent of the patients.[141] It appears as though garlic is effective in improving oxygen levels in the arterial blood and may help alleviate breathing issues. It is not effective in all patients, however, but it is certainly worth a try.

HEALTH

WELLNESS

PESTS

OTHER

72. SNAKEBITES

Venomous snakes are found throughout the world and can be a threat to humans, particularly in rural areas where they are more abundant. The majority of snakes are not poisonous but can still pack a powerful punch with their bite. If you are living in an area where snakes dwell, it is important to take precautions to prevent accidentally getting bitten. Always check pools and lakes before diving in to make sure you're not sharing the water with a snake or two. Keep hands and feet out of crevices, and avoid walking through tall grass. If hiking, wear close-toed shoes. Above all, leave snakes alone. Most snakebites are provoked by the person bitten. If bitten, remain still and seek medical attention immediately. You will see puncture marks around the wound and likely notice redness, swelling, and pain. Depending on the snake, you may also experience nausea, sweating, trouble seeing, or tingling in the limbs.

Always try to remember what the snake looked like in order to tell medical professionals that information so they can administer the correct antivenom, if needed. If the bite is from a nonpoisonous garter snake or a pet snake and the wound is clean and not too deep, initial treatment can begin at home.

Clean the wound with warm, fresh water and mild soap. Gently blot dry. Then consume garlic. Its antimicrobial and anti-inflammatory properties can reduce inflammation, pain, and the risk of secondary infection. Garlic was recommended to treat snakebites two thousand years ago by Pedanius Dioscorides, a Greek physician who wrote a five-volume encyclopedia on the medicinal use of plants. It was widely regarded as the leading authority in this area for 1500 years. Ayurvedic medicine also recommends garlic for snakebites and suggests consuming it with wine or ghee. Continue with garlic treatment until symptoms have disappeared. In the meantime, be sure to pay a visit to your doctor just to make sure the body is healing properly.

73. STOMACH ULCERS

Ulcers are holes in the protective lining of the stomach, small intestine, and esophagus. Sores develop that may cause stomach pain, bloating, heartburn, nausea, and fatty-food intolerance. Infection with *H. pylori* is thought to be the main cause. Overuse of painkillers, smoking, stress, and heavy alcohol use are other contributing factors. If *H. pylori* are present, treatment involves a course of antibiotics to kill the bacteria. Medications to neutralize, block, or reduce the production of stomach acid are often prescribed. It is imperative that the use of painkillers, cigarettes, and alcohol is greatly reduced or stopped.

The wide-spectrum antibiotic potential of garlic makes it useful as a therapeutic agent in resolving stomach ulcers caused by *H. pylori*. This was investigated, and results show that undiluted garlic oil, garlic powder, and allicin and diallyl trisulfide (both found in garlic) were all able to destroy *H. pylori* in a dose-dependent manner.[142] Even some antibiotic-resistant strains of *H. pylori* are susceptible to garlic.[143] One of the conventional drug treatments for stomach ulcers is omeprazole, a proton pump inhibitor. Consuming garlic along with this medicine showed a synergistic effect.[144] This may allow for a quicker resolution of *H. pylori* infections and a shorter course of treatment. Aged garlic extract was also comparable to omeprazole in protecting stomach tissues from changes generated by the formation of ulcers.[145]

74. SWIMMER'S EAR

Water that remains in the ear after swimming can cause an infection inside the outer ear canal. The warm, moist environment is the perfect breeding ground for bacteria or fungi that are commonly found in water or on the skin. They will readily invade the skin and multiply. The infection causes itching and redness, which can escalate to severe pain in and around the ear, discharge of pus, fever, and partial or complete blockage of the ear canal. To stop the infection, doctors commonly prescribe antibiotics, antifungals, or eardrops that contain both of these and steroids. Taking over-the-counter pain medications such as ibuprofen is also recommended.

An effective method of resolving swimmer's ear is to use garlic and olive oil. Peel a clove of garlic and cut it into several pieces. Heat a few tablespoons of olive oil in a double boiler on the stove over medium heat, and add the garlic. After twenty minutes, remove the boiler from the stove. Allow the garlic-infused oil to cool to a lukewarm temperature. Lay down with the infected ear facing up. Using a glass eyedropper or a cotton ball, transfer a few drops of the oil into the infected ear. Cover with a warm cloth. After ten minutes, sit upright and drain the ear of any oil. Repeat twice a day until the infection has cleared.

This works well whether the infection is bacterial or fungal. The most common fungi in swimmer's ear is *Aspergillus*. Concentrated garlic oil inhibited the growth of this fungi and had similar or better results than some pharmaceutical preparations.[146]

75. TOOTHACHE

Pain that is sharp or throbbing in or around a tooth is a toothache. The pain may be constant or only when pressure is applied to the tooth and is generally a result of the tooth's nerve root becoming irritated. Swelling around the tooth and headaches sometimes occur. Some causes are tooth decay, damaged fillings, infected gums, trauma to the tooth, or teeth grinding. Dental treatment is often necessary to fix a damaged tooth. Over-the-counter pain medications are used to temporarily dull pain and inflammation.

An alternative to medications like ibuprofen or acetaminophen is garlic. For severe pain, the most potent source of garlic is warranted—fresh, raw garlic. Peel a garlic clove and cut it in half. Press each cut side to either side of the tooth, making sure to cover the gums as well. This may cause a tingling or burning sensation. If it is uncomfortable, remove it and rinse the mouth with water. The garlic should bring down the swelling and reduce the pain. If an infection is causing the pain, garlic is an excellent antimicrobial and can reduce symptoms by killing the bacteria or fungi.

Another method is to crush several cloves of garlic and mix them with a teaspoon of sea salt. This paste can be applied directly to the affected tooth. After five minutes, rinse the mouth with salt water. A similar recipe using crushed garlic cloves, sea salt, and warm water can be used to make a mouth rinse. Swish this around the mouth for several minutes before spitting out. This can be done several times a day until the pain subsides.

76. WARTS

Warts are small skin growths caused by the human papillomavirus (HPV). They are usually flesh-colored and contain small black dots, which are actually clotted blood vessels. The hands and the fingers are the most common areas where they are found, which is not surprising since the virus is contagious. If warts occur on the soles of the feet, they are called plantar warts. Most warts go away on their own, but it may take a year or two. Many people find them embarrassing and opt to get rid of them using salicylic acid medications, freezing, or laser treatments. These methods can cause pain, blistering, and scarring.

An effective at-home treatment is garlic. This can be applied directly to the wart, with results expected within a month. Although this may seem like a long time, it is comparable or faster than over-the-counter medications. The usefulness of garlic was studied in fifty patients with recalcitrant multiple common warts. They were randomly assigned to use either a lipid garlic extract or saline on their warts. After one month, 96 percent of people using the lipid garlic extract saw complete resolution of their warts, with no recurrence. This was significantly different from the results in the saline group.[147] Garlic is thought to work by amplifying the immune response and reducing viral cells from multiplying.

Therefore garlic may be considered as a first line of treatment in wart removal or used when other methods have failed.

77. WEIGHT LOSS

When the body accumulates too much body fat, there is an increased risk of health problems like diabetes, heart disease, and certain cancers. Losing weight can improve or prevent any weight-induced conditions.

Fat accumulates on the body when more calories are eaten than burned. The body stores these excess calories as fat. Exercising and eating a healthy diet with appropriate calorie intake will help burn the stored fat and reduce body weight. During the weight-loss process, people often report reaching plateaus where they no longer seem to be able to continue losing weight despite continued efforts with exercise and dieting. This is because metabolism slows down as weight is lost.

Thermogenesis is one metabolic process that can be ramped up by eating garlic. Some of the sulfides in garlic increase thermogenesis, or heat production, in the cells of brown adipose tissue by elevating levels of adrenaline and noradrenaline, which are known to mobilize fat to burn for fuel.[148] This can lead to weight loss and was demonstrated in overweight subjects diagnosed with nonalcoholic fatty liver disease. Participants received either two garlic tablets or two placebo tablets a day. Those consuming garlic significantly reduced their body weight and body fat mass compared to the placebo group.[149]

HEALTH
WELLNESS
PESTS
OTHER

78. WOUND HEALING

Wounding the skin is a very common occurrence and happens to everyone. Whether it's slicing the tip of the finger while dicing carrots or slipping on gravel and scraping a knee, cuts and scrapes tear the skin tissue and often cause bleeding. If the wound is deep, bleeds heavily, or has an object embedded in it, seek medical attention. If it's minor, however, it can be addressed at home.

Wash your hands with soap and water. Clean the cut or scrape by pouring cool, clean water over it to remove dirt and debris. Then wash with soap and water. Once clean, an antibiotic ointment can be applied.

Aged garlic was observed to significantly improve wound healing in chickens. One-week-old chicks with dorsal wounds were topically exposed to differing concentrations of an aged garlic solution. All wounds exposed to garlic showed an increase in the movement of skin cells into the wounds, resulting in a decrease in the size of the wound. Collagen was laid down at a higher rate, and new blood vessels were abundantly formed. No significant changes were observed in the control group of chickens that did not receive the aged garlic solution.[150] Garlic as part of a honey-and-chitosan nanofiber wound dressing was even found to heal wounds faster than the commercial product Aquacel Ag, a commonly used sterile wound-dressing with silver.[151]

CHAPTER 3

EXPUNGE PESTS

79. ANTS

There are trillions of ants around the world, so it is no surprise to find them in your garden or home. These social insects live in large numbers, so if you see a few milling around some plants in the backyard or walking across the floor on the way to the pantry, beware. If allowed to go on their merry way, they will arrive in droves and make themselves at home.

There is no beneficial reason for ants to enter your home, but in the garden, they are helpful in aerating the soil for plants and in controlling some other insect populations. They also serve as food for lizards, birds, spiders, and other insects. However, that's pretty much where their usefulness ends. Ants can wreak havoc in the garden and will eat almost any fruit, vegetable, or plant. To make matters worse, they protect insects that produce honeydew (a sweet, sticky substance) and feed on plants, allowing these insects to thrive and potentially decimate your favorite greenery.

Ants are repelled by strong scents. Placing garlic in areas of the home where ants have been seen will ensure they don't return. Pay careful attention to sites of entry and be sure to place peeled and thickly sliced cloves of garlic at those places. When the garlic cloves have dried out, they can be removed and replaced with fresh garlic, if needed.

In the garden, you can spray ant colonies with a mixture of garlic and water. To create the spray, purée a few cloves of garlic in water and add to a spray bottle. This mixture can also be sprayed on the ant trail to disrupt the pheromones the ants leave to track their route. They will become confused and not find their way back to their feeding site.

....

80. BARBER POLE WORMS (IN ANIMALS)

This worm is a blood-sucking parasite that infests sheep and goats. It is a worldwide problem but tends to be more prevalent in temperate and sub-temperate regions, particularly when conditions are warm and wet. The larvae of the worm are eaten by sheep and goats during grazing and burrow into their stomachs. Here they develop into adults and feed on blood. If the infestation is large, the animals can bleed to death.

Naturally, livestock owners want to prevent an infestation, but keeping the worm population low is a challenge. Barber pole worms are prolific, and females can lay up to ten thousand eggs per day. These eggs are excreted in the feces of their host. They hatch into larvae and are ready to be consumed by another unsuspecting animal. Signs of an infestation include diarrhea, lethargy, anemia, growth retardation, edema, dehydration, and loss of milk production in lactating mothers.

Deworming drugs are used to try to control barber pole worm infestations, but they have little effectiveness because the worms are resistant to them. In areas where this parasite is common, sheep and goat owners can feed garlic to their livestock as part of their daily management practices. When garlic was orally fed to gerbils infected with barber pole worms, it reduced the parasitic burden in the gerbils by 68.7 percent. When combined with Mexican marigold, 87.5 percent of the worms were removed.[152] The strong larvicidal activity of garlic against the parasite suggests adding garlic to the feed of at-risk animals should prevent barber pole worms from thriving in their hosts.

81. DARKLING BEETLES

Darkling beetles are scavengers and decomposers. This may seem like a good thing for the garden. They'll clean up debris, dead plants, and rotting wood. But they will also feed on living plant material, too, and attack vegetables, fruits, seeds, and flowers. The larval stage of darkling beetles is the mealworm. These are pests, too, and are frequently found in the garden eating young plants or munching away in stored grains like cereal and flour.

Considering that there are thousands of different species of darkling beetles and that they can be found all over the world, you are likely to find them in your backyard garden. Depending on the species, the adults live from several months to ten years, and the females lay hundreds to thousands of eggs over their lifetime. That's a lot of destructive potential that needs to be harnessed.

All stages of the darkling beetle life cycle find garlic toxic. Garlic essential oil was applied topically to larvae, pupae, and adult insects. It was most harmful to the larvae, followed by the pupae and adults. Symptoms of intoxication, injury, and death followed within twenty to forty hours after exposure.[153] Garlic essential oil can also be used as a repellent. Ninety percent of larvae were driven away after twelve hours of exposure.[154] It appears that garlic essential oil can serve as an effective control agent for mealworms and darkling beetles.

PEST SPRAY

1 teaspoon garlic essential oil
1/4 cup castile soap
30 ounces water

1. Mix all ingredients in a 32-ounce spray bottle.
2. Spray directly on the mealworms and beetles.

82. EUROPEAN STARLINGS

Sixty European starlings were released into New York's Central Park in 1890, with forty more being released the next year. The population of these birds in North America has since exploded to over 200 million.

These birds travel and feed in flocks, so when they descend on a field, they can wreak excessive damage. They are a major pest to farmers and consume both wild and cultivated fruits and seeds. They even go so far as to pull sprouting grains to eat the seeds. Livestock are also affected. Starlings deplete livestock rations, selectively eating the high-protein supplements added to the feed. Farm animals are left deficient in nutrients and fail to thrive, forcing the farmer to purchase more costly supplements and feed.

A soft approach to deterring starling populations from settling in an area is to use garlic oil. After overnight food deprivation, European starlings were given the choice to either eat garlic

HEALTH

WELLNESS

PESTS

OTHER

oil–impregnated granules or go hungry. They significantly reduced their consumption by 61 to 65 percent.[155] Garlic oil repels these birds, so putting some garlic oil granules strategically around farmer's fields and feedlots may be enough to send the starlings away in search of more palatable food.

83. MOLES

Moles are underground-dwelling mammals that typically feed on insects, worms, and other arthropods living in the ground. Plants and seeds constitute only a small percentage of their diet, but they are still very harmful to lawns and gardens due to the tunnels they dig.

Some of the tunnels are shallow and look like tubes running just underneath the grass. However, extensive damage can be done very quickly since the tunnels are dug at a rate of six meters an hour. Mounds of dirt that look like mini volcanos may also be evident. These indicate mole feeding sites. Other tunnels go as deep as ten inches and serve as the main highway through which the moles travel from their dens underground to their feeding areas near the surface.

Typical repellents include sonic, ultrasonic, and electronic vibrations. These may work but can be expensive and require maintenance. Chemical repellents are also used, but these also have their drawbacks. They may not be safe for pets, children, wildlife, or other plants. Trapping and relocating moles is an effective way to remove them from an area. It often requires the help of a professional who can humanely trap and move the mole to a place where it will thrive but not become a pest for another landowner.

An inexpensive method to deter moles from lawns and gardens is to use garlic. Moles have a highly developed sense of smell, so strong odors, like those from garlic, are offensive to them. They will leave the area to avoid the smell. Whole peeled garlic cloves or crushed garlic can be put into the tunnels and mounds. The moles will abandon these tunnels and build new ones, hopefully far away. If they continue to dig in the area, maintain this practice until they have moved on. Spraying garlic water over the soil of their feeding sites will also encourage them to leave.

GARLIC-WATER REPELLENT

1 gallon water
5–6 minced garlic cloves

1. Boil the water on the stove. Turn off the heat and add the garlic cloves. Allow the garlic to infuse the water for about 20 minutes.
2. Remove from the stove and strain the minced garlic out of the water. Transfer the water to a spray bottle. Spray the soil on the mounds and tunnel openings with the water.

84. MOSQUITOS

Mosquitos are hardy pests that have been around for millions of years. They are tough to get rid of and even tougher to avoid when outside. The females bite humans in order to use their blood to develop their eggs. As they do, they inject saliva into the skin, which can cause an immune system response. The results are tiny red spots in some people or itchy, swollen, red welts in others.

HEALTH

WELLNESS

PESTS

OTHER

Mosquitos can smell their prey from up to fifty meters away and are attracted to carbon dioxide, movement, chemicals in sweat, and heat. Getting bitten by a mosquito may not seem like such a big deal, but these pesky insects can carry diseases like West Nile virus, Zika virus, malaria, and yellow fever. To avoid getting bitten, many people use chemical repellent sprays or lotions on their skin. To avoid direct application to the skin, some people use chemical repellent paper strips worn on the body or placed in an outdoor area.

Many people want to avoid chemical-based repellents and are turning to natural products as alternatives. Garlic wards off several species of mosquitos known to carry diseases like the West Nile virus, encephalitis, and dengue fever.

Toxic sugar baits containing microencapsulated garlic oil or microencapsulated garlic oil plus a 1 percent boric acid solution were used to attract two types of mosquitos known for carrying West Nile Virus and/or inducing encephalitis, an infection causing inflammation of the brain. After two days, the mortality rate was 86 and 91 percent for the two species of mosquitos feeding on the garlic-oil sugar baits, while the garlic-oil plus boric-acid baits generated fatality rates of 91 and 99 percent.[156]

Another study using microencapsulated garlic-oil sugar baits corroborates garlic's efficacy, this time on the Asian tiger mosquito, a known carrier of dengue fever. Gardens with high numbers of these mosquitos had their perimeters sprayed with the garlic-oil bait. The entire mosquito population collapsed after about four days and continued to decline. After twenty-six days, only 15 percent of the original mosquito population remained.[157] Garlic can be safely used to reduce mosquito numbers and the risk of infection and disease.

85. POWDERY MILDEW

This fungal disease is commonly found on outdoor garden plants and usually appears later in the growing season. It attacks young leaves and covers them with a white or gray powder, usually on the upper surface. The leaves curl inward and may turn brown and fall from the plant. Unopened flower buds covered in powdery mildew have stunted growth and fail to open. The fungal spores can overwinter on plants or in the soil and be transferred from one plant to another by wind, insects, or water. It is not just flowering plants but varieties of vegetables that are susceptible to this fungus, including tomatoes, beans, and squash. Fungicides can be used to treat this infection. If the plant is indoors, sulfur prills burned into dust and layered over the leaves will work. This changes the pH of the leaves and inhibits the growth of powdery mildew.

Instead of using toxic chemicals or an expensive sulfur burner, you can use a garlic spray to stop the growth and spread of powdery mildew. Spray directly on the leaves of plants infected with powdery mildew. The soil around the base of the plants should be sprayed as well. This prevents viable fungal spores from splashing onto the plant when it rains. Both the garlic and neem oil have fungicidal properties and will dispose of the powdery mildew quickly. The dish detergent acts as an emulsifier to keep the product well mixed, although a quick shake of the bottle before use is recommended.

GARLIC FUNGAL SPRAY

1 liter garlic-water repellent (see page 105)
1 teaspoon neem oil
1 squirt dish detergent

Combine the garlic water, neem oil, and dish detergent in a spray bottle. Shake and use.

86. SCAB DISEASE

The plant fungus known as scab disease can affect fruit, vegetables, and ornamental flowering plants. It can look like an overgrowth of tissue on the leaves, stems, tubers, and fruits, much like a scab covering a wound. The crustaceous lesions that result form spots on the surface of leaves and on the flesh of fruit. As the infection matures, the leaves develop holes, curl, and drop early. The fruit develops rot deep within, inhibiting growth and making them inedible. This infection can be introduced into a crop field from sowing infected seeds or through spores carried in by wind, water, or field workers. Once scab is present, it can survive the winter and be difficult to get rid of. It can occur season after season if fungal management practices are not implemented. Several commercial fungicides are registered for use against scab.

Regular sprays with garlic during the growing season can keep scab from destroying plants and fruits.[158] Using either the plain garlic water recipe (see page 105) or the garlic fungal spray recipe (see previous section) can kill the fungus responsible for the infection. This method prevents the use of harmful chemicals that can affect other plants, beneficial insects, pets, and even children.

87. SNAKES

Snakes are an important part of the ecosystem, keeping mice, birds, frogs, insects, grubs, and other pests at bay. Unfortunately, many people are uncomfortable or squeamish around snakes, even though most pose no threat to them. The majority of snakes are nonvenomous and actively avoid encounters with humans, but it's important to know the harmful snakes living in your area. An accidental encounter can lead to a painful bite, which can result in a secondary infection. It can even be life threatening, particularly to children and pets.

Keeping snakes out of the yard and away from the home is a concern for many. Snakes like to hide in tall grass, wood piles, and overgrown vegetation. Removing these will force snakes to relocate. Make sure to seal all openings into the home, garage, and outbuildings because snakes have a way of finding openings and will move indoors in search of food or to set up a nesting site. If a snake does take up residence in the home or yard, an expert can be called in to safely and humanely remove it. There are also snake traps that can be used indoors. When caught, relocate the snake to another suitable habitat.

To avoid dealing with this problem in the first place, you can use garlic to deter snakes from entering your property. Mix equal amounts of crushed garlic and rock salt. Drop some of this paste around snake nesting areas. Spraying garlic water (see page 105) around windows, doors, crawl spaces, or the perimeter of the home and property should also repel snakes and force them to find more pleasing habitats. If it rains, be sure to reapply the paste or spray.

88. SPIDER MITES

There are many species of spider mites, and they are very destructive to both indoor and outdoor plants. One of the most common ones is the two-spotted spider mite. This arachnid is tiny, only 1/50th of an inch long. It lives in a colony and has been reported to infest over two hundred species of plants, including trees, ornamental plants, vegetables, and fruits. The eggs overwinter on the vegetation. When the temperatures rise, the eggs hatch, and mite numbers can explode exponentially within weeks. They feed on plants by penetrating the plant tissue with their needle-like, piercing mouth. The damage produces yellow or white spots all over the leaves. The leaves eventually turn yellow or copper and fall off. Flowers brown and wither. Severe or prolonged spider mite infestations kill the plant.

To control populations, water can be used to spray the plants to dislodge some of the mites. This only removes a portion of the mites, though, and they can quickly replenish their numbers. Other insects can be introduced to prey on the spider mites. This is effective under the right conditions, but the end result is difficult to predict. Insecticides destroy spider mites, but many of these affect the plant, other insect populations, or surrounding vegetation. Use insecticides judiciously and consider low-impact or organic alternatives.

Garlic naturally repels the two-spotted spider mite. These mites infest strawberry plants and can ravage entire crops. Garlic intercropped with strawberry plants reduced the two-spotted spider mite numbers on strawberry plants by 52 percent. The number of eggs on the plants were 64 percent less than the number of eggs on plants without garlic intercropping. The more rows of garlic in between the strawberry rows, the greater the spider mite repellency.[159] Consider planting garlic in the garden or add to the landscaping around the house if spider mites are a concern.

89. SPIDERS

There are tens of thousands of species of spiders throughout the world. In North America, only a few have bites that are harmful to humans. These are the brown recluse, widows, hobo, and yellow sac spiders. Most, however, are harmless to humans and provide a valuable service for us: they eat other insects that can be found in the home, like earwigs, roaches, mosquitos, flies, ants, and other crawling or flying pests.

Despite their usefulness, it's not good to have too many spiders in the home. Females lay eggs in a sac or cocoon and attach them to their web or carry them around. One female can lay hundreds of eggs, so when these hatch, an infestation inside the house is likely. One spider tucked into a darkened corner or a few hidden from sight are fine, but when they are highly visible at every turn, it's time to get rid of them.

Vacuum regularly to remove webs and egg sacs. Take care to keep other insects out of the house so spiders have nothing to eat. Make your home a less desirable habitat by removing clutter and drying out damp areas like basements. As a final step, place repellents around the home to send spiders packing.

Spiders don't like the smell of garlic. Spray garlic water (see page 105) where you have noticed spiders or where webs are present.

Pay attention to doors and windows, which are potential areas of entry—you don't want more coming in after you have gotten rid of the previous ones. A few drops of peppermint essential oil can be added to the garlic water. Peppermint repels spiders, too, and the scent can help mask the odor of garlic to human noses.

90. TAPEWORMS

Tapeworms are intestinal parasites that infect animals and humans. Eating contaminated food or water containing microscopic tapeworm eggs or larval cysts or coming into contact with infested soil and touching your mouth is a sure way to get tapeworms. If eggs are ingested, they develop into larvae in the intestines and then move to other tissues, usually the liver and lungs, and develop into cysts. They can grow up to fifty feet long and live more than twenty years. Many people with intestinal infections don't have any symptoms. Others experience nausea, diarrhea, weakness, weight loss, and abdominal pain. If cysts have developed in other organs of the body, the person may develop a fever, cystic lumps, or allergic reactions. Seizures have even happened with severe infections. Once diagnosed, oral medications to kill adult tapeworms are prescribed. If cysts have formed, they may need to be drained or removed by surgery.

Spillage of live larvae during surgical removal of tapeworm cysts is a major cause of tapeworm recurrence. To prevent this from happening, when cysts are surgically removed, doctors often inject the cysts with medication to destroy the larvae. But, currently, there is no medication for tapeworm cysts that is both safe and effective. Garlic flowers have been discovered to kill tapeworm larvae in cysts and can be used to stop further growth and prevent reinfection during surgery. Tapeworm larvae from cysts found in sheep livers were exposed to different concentrations of garlic flowers. After ten minutes of the higher concentration, 67 percent of the larvae were killed, and after 180 minutes, 98 percent died.[160] Extract of garlic flowers appears to be a potent destroyer of tapeworm larvae and can be used to greatly reduce the risk of recurrence in humans undergoing tapeworm cyst removal surgery.

91. TICKS

These parasitic pests feed on the blood of other animals, and their bite can spread disease. There are over 900 species of ticks throughout the world. In North America, the deer tick has been getting a lot of attention for its role in transmitting Lyme disease. Deer ticks are small, about 1/8 of an inch, and can vary in color from reddish brown to blueish gray. They blend in to the environment and often go unnoticed. When they sense a host is approaching, they scramble up shrubbery, grass, or trees and grab onto the host as it brushes by them. They crawl around the host until they find a good place to feed and deeply embed their mouthparts into the skin; there they remain for days, feeding on blood. Because their bites are painless, most people don't realize they've been bitten. After walking through woods or hiking in tall grass, be sure to check your body for ticks. Don't forget about any pets; ticks love them too.

Taking care to eliminate ticks from your property will greatly decrease the chances of being bitten by a tick. While most bites are not serious, some ticks do carry disease that they pass onto people and animals. In addition, the wound created by the bite may become infected. Keeping lawns mowed and yards clear of debris can limit areas for ticks to inhabit. Spraying pesticides around the perimeter of the property is also a popular method to keep ticks away. While this can be effective, pesticides can cause damage to other forms of life, both above and below ground. Garlic used as a natural spray can repel ticks and not harm other wildlife or the environment. A garlic juice spray was used in Connecticut over a three-year period to determine its ability to control the population of the nymphal stage of deer ticks. This stage of the tick is more likely to go unnoticed and transmit Lyme disease because of its smaller size. Up to a 59 percent reduction of tick numbers were noted during the post-spray period. Multiple applications were needed, but it looks like garlic can be used to decrease tick numbers around the home and yard.[161]

CHAPTER 4

....

EMPLOY EXTRAORDINARY USES

....

92. APHRODISIAC

The term *aphrodisiac* originated from Aphrodite, the Greek goddess of love. Over the centuries, plant and animal products have been used to increase sexual desire and, in turn, enhance sexual performance and pleasure. The natural aphrodisiac inherent in our physical makeup are pheromones, chemicals emitted by the body whose scent subconsciously attracts others by triggering physiological and behavioral responses. These can be supplemented with foods and other agents to increase desire and attraction.

Garlic is said to be a potent aphrodisiac and has been used for centuries to increase libido. It's fair to say that if used as an aphrodisiac, both individuals should partake. Garlic causes a strong odor on the breath, but it is much less noticeable in others if your own breath is garlicky. To make the situation more palatable, consume mint leaves, raw lettuce leaves, or raw apples[162] after eating garlic to neutralize the odor-causing compounds.

Perhaps garlic's reputation stems from a more physiological effect. Men with atherosclerosis have plaque clogging their arteries. This reduces blood flow, including blood flow to the penis, and weakens erections. Men consuming high doses of garlic powder reduced their plaque volume by up to 18 percent.[163] Blood can now flow more rapidly and easily to areas where it's needed. High blood pressure also affects the quality of erections. It changes the elasticity of the blood vessels so that blood will flow into the penis slower and leave quicker than usual. Garlic can help by lowering both systolic and diastolic blood pressure.[164]

HEALTH

WELLNESS

PESTS

OTHER

93. DISINFECTING SPRAY

There is a plethora of products touted as cleaning agents to destroy germs and grime and make countertops, sinks, and windows shine. Miraculous claims aside, since there are no US federal regulations for chemicals in household products, many may contain toxic compounds that can harm your health and the environment. Some contain known carcinogens, formaldehyde, and other highly toxic compounds known to cause reproductive, neurotoxic, and respiratory damage. These chemicals can build up in our bodies over time and trigger disease. When the instructions for use include wearing safety goggles and gloves and state that inhalation could be harmful or fatal, you would do well to avoid them. Only 7 percent of cleaning products list all their ingredients; even if products that claim to be natural or green, they can still be toxic, so beware of these too.

A simple, non-toxic disinfecting spray can be made at home with a short list of commonly available ingredients. It is safe for you, your family, your pets, and the environment. This solution will destroy germs and wash away dirt and residue on surfaces. It can be used on cutting boards, countertops (but not marble or granite), windows, sinks, microwaves, tile, and stainless steel.

DISINFECTING SPRAY

1 cup water
1 cup apple cider vinegar
6 roughly chopped garlic cloves
20 drops wild orange, eucalyptus, or lavender essential oil (optional)

1. Combine the water, apple cider vinegar, and garlic cloves. Add the essential oil, if desired. This will boost cleaning and disinfecting power and improve the aroma.
2. Let it sit for about an hour before using. Spray on surfaces and wipe off with a clean microfiber cloth.

94. FISHING BAIT AND LURES

Fishing can be a job, a hobby, or a bonding experience shared among friends. It can provide food or simply a means to unwind and relax. For most, the end goal is to catch as many fish as possible (or allowed), and for this, proper bait is needed. Good baits will lure fish into biting the hook, but different fish prefer different baits. Natural or live baits are effective ways to catch fish because of their familiar odor, texture, and color. Worms are one of the best-known and most universal live baits. Leeches and minnows are also used with success and can be purchased in a bait shop. To save money, try collecting snails, mussels, clams, or insects like beetles and caterpillars to use—fish love those as well. Another option is to use an artificial lure. There are hundreds to choose from. They are made to look attractive to fish, and their movements, colors, and shapes imitate prey.

Both kinds of lures have their drawbacks: artificial lures can be expensive, and handling natural, live bait is not for the squeamish. Garlic is an unusual alternative recommended by some fishermen because fish are highly attracted to the strong odor. There are even a number of garlic-oil products marketed as sprays for bait and lures. They are supposed to be very effective on trout, steelhead, and salmon. Some artificial lures even have garlic odor permeated through the soft plastic. Garlic also masks the human odors left on the lures after handling. If you want to make your own garlic fish-attractants at home, try the recipes below.

GARLIC SPRAY FOR FISH LURES

1/2 cup olive oil
1/4 cup garlic powder

1. Mix the two ingredients in a jar to create a slurry.
2. Soft plastic lures can be soaked for a few hours in this before heading out to fish, or the slurry can be transferred to a spray bottle, sprayed on the lures, and allowed to dry.

GARLIC BAIT

1 tablespoon petroleum jelly
1 teaspoon garlic powder

1. Mix the two ingredients thoroughly.
2. Spread a thin layer over the bait (or lure) prior to fishing.

95. FIX CRACKED GLASS

Hairline cracks in windows, shower doors, tabletops, or mirrors begin as small, thin, vein-like lines that can spread and deepen over time. Cracked glass can cut the skin if touched and can shatter if pressure is applied. It poses a safety issue in the home and should be rectified immediately. Garlic can be used to stabilize cracks in glass and prevent them from spreading.

Crush a garlic clove and rub the sticky, viscous liquid directly over the crack. Apply to both sides of the glass if the crack has penetrated the entire depth. Allow to dry, and reapply if needed. The garlic juice will adhere the two sides of the glass together and prevent or slow further damage.

96. GIFT TOPPER

Gift-giving happens throughout the year to commemorate special occasions, personal achievements, or just about any other event that warrants recognition. A beautifully wrapped gift shows the care and effort taken in choosing the right gift for its intended, particularly when the design is handcrafted and unique.

Rather than adding a bow on top of the present, artfully arrange two to three young garlic heads together and tie the stems with twine to secure them in place. This organic touch works wonderfully with burlap, canvas, linen, or brown paper wrapping. Finally, add a few sprigs of fresh herbs to the garlic-head topper to bring a pop of color and a muslin-fabric personalized gift tag to complete the look.

97. GLUE

Glues have been used for thousands of years: they have been found in ancient products from Egyptian wood furniture to Roman and

Greek tile floors. Ancient glues were derived from organic com-pounds with sticky properties that can hold surfaces together. The earliest glues were made with collagen extracted from skin, bones, and other connective tissue. Later, other tacky animal proteins like casein from milk and albumin from blood were discovered. Plants have adhesive compounds too. Agar, algin, and gum arabic are a few that have been extracted from plants and used to make glue. Centuries ago, Italian painters used garlic as a gluing agent in their wall and easel paintings.[165] Today, glue is used in countless appli-cations and has even found a place in the medical world, replacing stitches to close wounds.

Glue can be easily purchased and is relatively inexpensive, but the glues most commonly used at home are often petroleum- or solvent-based, with a plethora of harmful chemicals that can cause skin and respiratory irritation. To avoid these issues, simple garlic glue can be made by crushing a garlic clove and using the juice. It works wonderfully on paper, so if an old envelope has lost its stick-iness, add garlic juice to seal it. Children especially would benefit from using this eco-friendly glue in their art projects. Parents can let them freely work without fear of adverse reactions from harm-ful toxins.

98. HOLIDAY AND FESTIVAL DECORATIONS

Holidays and festivals throughout the year are a time of celebra-tion, of gathering with family and friends to acknowledge tradition, religion, people, and events. Each has its own themed decorations with unique color combinations like red and green for Christmas and orange and black for Halloween. It can be refreshing to have new decorations to put out rather than the same ones year after year. This is particularly true if they are homemade and unique. Garlic bulbs are the perfect starting point to create cute and fun accessories to complement the day.

For Valentine's Day, paint two entire bulbs red. Add googly eyes to each, then draw eyelashes on one and smiles on both. Display this cute pair on a table where they can be easily viewed. Similar decorations can be made for other celebrations. For Christmas, make garlic-bulb elf faces with paint and markers. Be creative and add felt cone-shaped hats or ears. For Halloween, bulbs can be painted orange and the tip of the stem painted green. Use a black marker to draw a face on the garlic "pumpkin." These decorations can only be used for the current year and should not be stored in the hopes of displaying them again next year. New ones will have to be made, but that's half the fun!

99. SEASICKNESS

Motion sickness is something most everyone has experienced at some point in their lives. Sea excursions in high winds and choppy water create up-and-down, side-to-side, circular, and jerky movements, resulting in severe dizziness, cold sweats, nausea, and vomiting for some. It happens when the signals received from the eyes, the body, and the inner ear send conflicting messages to the brain. Medications are often prescribed in pill or patch form but can cause drowsiness, dry mouth, blurred vision, and disorientation.

A natural preventative to seasickness is to chew garlic cloves before and during the trip. It's important to begin this process beforehand. Taking garlic once nausea begins likely won't help. This solution may be more appropriate for those sailing on smaller crafts with family and friends who won't mind your garlic breath as much, knowing that it is preventing you from feeling sick. On larger boats filled with many strangers, however, they may not be as forgiving and might steer clear of you. On the bright side, you'll be given lots of personal space to enjoy the scenery.

100. SPLINTERS

Splinters are slivers of material from wood, metal, glass, or anything else that can break into sharp fragments and penetrate the skin. Common situations in which you might get splinters are when walking barefoot across a wooden deck or cleaning up broken glass. Splinters are painful and may bleed. Often, they are visible under the skin, but some splinters are embedded deep within the tissue and need a doctor to remove them.

Shallow splinters can be removed at home with tweezers. Grip the end of the splinter with the tweezers and pull gently in the opposite direction from which the fragment entered the skin. If this doesn't work, or if a piece of the sliver is still under the skin, another method is needed.

Apply a thin layer of a carrier oil like almond or jojoba oil to protect the skin. Layer with a slice of raw garlic. Secure the garlic in place with duct tape or a bandage. After a few hours, check under the garlic. Don't worry if the splinter hasn't emerged yet:

each person's reaction time is unique. But eventually, the splinter should work its way out of the skin. Once the splinter has surfaced, gently remove it with tweezers. Some people are sensitive to raw garlic on the skin and may experience a burning sensation. If this is the case, do not use this method.

101. WREATHS

The appearance of wreaths throughout history gives a glimpse into the culture and tradition of the times. Greeks and Romans made ring-shaped wreaths using twigs, fruits, flowers, and leaves. They were worn on the head and represented status, occupation, rank, or other achievements. Today, laurel wreaths are given to graduating students across the world to represent their academic success. Wreaths are also prominent in Christian history. Advent wreaths made of evergreen branches and four candles reminded the faithful to commemorate the birth of Jesus and prepare for his eventual return. The hanging of Christmas wreaths has become a tradition in many homes. While most still use fresh evergreens, wreath designs have become elaborate and colorful. Today, the displaying of wreaths encompasses just about any special occasion and can be placed anywhere in the house. They are made from natural and artificial greenery, an array of fabrics, fruits, flowers, or berries, and anything else that can be found in a craft store. Some are small and can be used as candle rings, while others are large and can be hung over the fireplace. They can be elegant or old fashioned, casual or formal. No matter what the style, wreaths are a popular décor to fit any affair.

Natural elements in a wreath embody a fresh, organic, at-home feel. Garlic can be artfully arranged in wreaths to visually add light, shape, and texture and balance out the use of artificial pieces. It can also be used alone to create a wreath entirely of garlic.

SIMPLE GARLIC WREATH

12-inch wire ring
newspaper
binding wire
stub wires
garlic bulbs

1. Crunch the newspaper into crinkly lengths and wrap it around and around the wire ring until the ring is completely covered.
2. Secure the paper in place by repeating the process with the binding wire. Make sure to twist the two ends of the wire together when they meet to ensure it stays in place.
3. Next, pierce the center of three garlic bulbs with stub wire. Leave a few inches of wire at both ends. Lay the bulbs across the wire wreath frame and tightly wrap the ends of the wire together behind the frame.
4. Repeat this process until the full circle of the wreath is adorned with garlic bulbs. Try to layer the smaller bulbs on the inside and the larger ones on the outside. This makes for a more uniform look.

Note: This wreath will initially smell strongly of garlic, but that will fade over time. To avoid this, simply use glue instead of wire to secure the bulbs onto the frame.

NOTES

1. Mirondo, Rita, and Sheryl Barringer. 2016. "Deodorization of garlic breath by foods, and the role of polyphenol oxidase and phenolic compounds." *Journal of Food Science* 81 (10): C2425–C2430.
2. Koch, H. P., and L. D. Lawson. *Garlic: The Science and Therapeutic Application of* Allium sativum *L. and Related Species*. New York, New York: Williams and Wilkins, 1996.
3. Moyers, S. B. *Garlic in Health, History, and World Cuisine*. St. Petersburg, Florida: Suncoast Press, 1996.
4. Lawson, L. D., and R. Bauer. *Phytomedicines of Europe: Chemistry and Biological Activity*. Washington, DC. ACS Symposium Series 691, American Chemical Society, 1998. 176–209.
5. Moyers, S. B., *Garlic in Health, History, and World Cuisine*.
6. Green, O. C., and N. G. Polydoris. "The chemistry of garlic and onions." *Garlic, Cancer and Heart Disease: Review and Recommendations*. Chicago, Illinois: GN Communications, 1993. 21–41.
7. Riddle, J. M. "The medicines of Greco-Roman antiquity as a source of medicines for today." *Prospecting for Drugs in Ancient and Medieval European Texts: A Scientific Approach*. Amsterdam, The Netherlands: Harwood Academic Publishers, 1996. 7–17.
8. Koch, H. P., et al., *Garlic: The Science and Therapeutic Application of* Allium sativum *L. and Related Species*.
9. Ibid.
10. Bergner, P. *The Healing Power of Garlic*. Rocklin, California: Prima Publishing, 1996. 3–26.
11. Moyers, S. B., *Garlic in Health, History, and World Cuisine*.
12. Hajheydari, Z., M. Jamshidi, J. Akbari, and R. Mohammadpour. 2007. "Combination of topical garlic gel and betamethasone valerate cream in the treatment of localized alopecia areata: a double-blind randomized controlled study." *Indian Journal of Dermatology, Venereology and Leprology* 73: 29–32.
13. Nillert N., W. Pannangrong, J. U. Welbat, W. Chaijaroonkhanarak, K. Sripanidkulchai, and B. Sripanidkulchai. 2017. "Neuroprotective effects of aged garlic extract on cognitive dysfunction and neuroinflammation induced by β-amyloid in rats." *Nutrients* 39 (1): 24.

14. Chauhan, N. B. and J. Sandoval. 2007. "Amelioration of early cognitive deficits by aged garlic extract in Alzheimer's transgenic mice." *Phytotherapy Research* 21 (7): 629–640.

15. Shin, I. S., J. Hong, C. M. Jeon, N. R. Shin, O. K. Kwon, H. S. Kim, J. C. Kim, S. R. Oh, and K. S. Ahn. 2013. "Diallyl-disulfide, an organosulfur compound of garlic, attenuates airway inflammation via activation of the Nrf-2/HO-1 pathway and NF-kappaB suppression." *Food and Chemical Toxicology* 62: 506–513.

16. Zare, A., P. Farzaneh, Z. Pourpak, F. Zahedi, M. Moin, S. Shahabi, and Z. M. Hassan. 2008. "Purified aged garlic extract modulates allergic airway inflammation in BALB/c mice." *Iran Journal of Allergy Asthma and Immunology* 7 (3): 133–141.

17. Ide, N., and B. H. Lau. 1997. "Garlic compounds protect vascular endothelial cells from oxidized low density lipoprotein–induced injury." *Journal of Pharmacy and Pharmacology* 49: 908–911.

18. Koscielny, J., D. Klussendorf, R. Latza, R. Schmitt, H. Radtke, G. Siegel, and H. Kiesewetter. 1999. "The antiatherosclerotic effect of *Allium sativum*." *Atherosclerosis* 144: 237–249.

19. Breithaupt-Grogler, K., M. Ling, H. Boudoulas, and G. G. Belz. 1997. "Protective effect of chronic garlic intake on elastic properties of aorta in the elderly." *Circulation* 96: 2649–2655.

20. Ledezma, E., L. DeSousa, A. Jorquera, J. Sanchez, A. Lander, E. Rodriguez, M. K. Jain, and R. Apitz-Castro. 1996. "Efficacy of ajoene, an organosulphur derived from garlic, in the short-term therapy of tinea pedis." *Mycoses* 39 (9–10): 393–395.

21. Ledezma, E., K. Marcano, and A. Jorquera. 2000. "Efficacy of ajoene in the treatment of tinea pedis: A double-blind and comparative study with terbinafine." *Journal of the American Academy of Dermatology* 43: 829–832.

22. Harris, J. C., S. Plummer, M. P. Turner, and D. Lloyd. 2000. "The microaerophilic flagellate *Giardia intestinalis: Allium sativum* (garlic) is an effective antigiardial." *Microbiology* 146 (12): 3119–3127.

23. Ankri, S., and D. Mirelman. 1999. "Antimicrobial properties of allicin from garlic." *Microbes and Infection* 1 (2): 125–129.

24. Bespalov, V. G., N. Barash, O. A. Ivanova, P. Krzhivitskiĭ, V. F. Semiglazov, V. A. Aleksandrov, N. A. Sobenin, and A. N. Orekhov AN. 2004. "Study of an antioxidant dietary supplement 'Karinat' in patients with benign breast disease." *Voprosy Onkologii* 50 (4): 467–472.

25. Lamm, D., and D. R. Riggs. 2000. "The potential application of *Allium sativum* (garlic) for the treatment of bladder cancer." *Urologic Clinics North America* 27: 157–162.

26. Shin, D.Y., H. J. Cha, G. Y. Kim, W. J. Kim, and Y. H. Choi. 2013. "Inhibiting invasion into human bladder carcinoma 5637 cells with diallyl trisulfide by inhibiting matrix metalloproteinase activities and tightening tight junctions." *International Journal of Molecular Science* 14 (10): 19911–19922.

27. Kim, W. T., S. P. Seo, Y. J. Byun, H. W. Kang, Y. J. Kim, S. C. Lee, P. Jeong, Y. Seo, S. Y. Choe, D. J. Kim, S. K. Kim, S. K. Moon, Y. H. Choi, G. T. Lee, I. Y. Kim, S. J. Yun, and W. J. Kim. 2017. "Garlic extract in bladder cancer prevention: evidence from T24 bladder cancer cell xenograft model, tissue microarray, and gene network analysis." *International Journal of Oncology* 51 (1): 204–212.

28. Roseblade, A., A. Ung, and M. Bebawy. 2017. "Synthesis and in vitro biological evaluation of thiosulfinate derivatives for the treatment of human multi-drug-resistant breast cancer." *Acta Pharmacologia Sinica* 38 (10): 1353–1368.

29. Sigounas, G., "S-allylmercaptocysteine inhibits cell proliferation and reduces the viability of erythroleukemia, breast, and prostate cancer cell lines."

30. Pourzand, A., A. Tajaddini, S. Pirouzpanah, M. Asghari-Jafarabadi, N. Samadi, A. R. Ostadrahimi, and Z. Sanaat. 2016. "Associations between dietary allium vegetables and risk of breast cancer: a hospital-based matched case-control study." *Journal of Breast Cancer* 19 (3): 292–300.

31. Josling, P. 2001. "Preventing the common cold with a garlic supplement: a double-blind, placebo-controlled survey." *Advances in Therapy* 18 (4): 189–193.

32. Yousuf, S., A. Ahmad, A. Khan, N. Manzoor, and L. A. Khan. 2010. "Effect of diallyldisulphide on an antioxidant enzyme system in *Candida* species." *Canadian Journal of Microbiology* 56 (10): 816–821.

33. Khodavandi, A., F. Alizadeh, N. S. Harmal, S. M. Sidik, F. Othman, Z. Sekawi, M. A. Jahromi, K. P. Ng, and P. P. Chong. 2011. "Comparison between efficacy of allicin and fluconazole against *Candida albicans in vitro* and in a systemic candidiasis mouse model." *FEMS Microbiology Letters* 315 (2): 87–93.

34. Urbina, J. A., E. Marchan, K. Lazardi, G. Visbal, R. Apitz-Castro, F. Gil, T. Aguirre, M. M. Piras, and R. Piras. 1993. "Inhibition of phosphatidylcholine biosynthesis and cell proliferation in *Trypanosoma cruzi* by ajoene, an anti-platelet compound isolated from garlic." *Biochemical Pharmacology* 45 (12): 2381–2387.

35. Tanaka, S., K. Haruma, M. Yoshihara, G. Kajiyama, K. Kira, H. Amagase, and K. Chayama. 2006. "Aged garlic extract has potential suppressive effect on colorectal adenomas in humans." *Journal of Nutrition* 136 (3): 821S–826S.

36. Ngo, S. N., D. B. Williams, L. Cobiac, and R. J. Head. 2007. "Does garlic reduce risk of colorectal cancer? A systematic review." *Journal of Nutrition* 137 (10): 2264–2269.

37. Bjarnsholt, T., P. Ø. Jensen, T. B. Rasmussen, L. Christophersen, H. Calum, M. Hentzer, H. P. Hougen, J. Rygaard, C. Moser, L. Eberl, N. Høiby, and M. Givskov. 2005. "Garlic blocks quorum sensing and promotes rapid clearing of pulmonary *Pseudomonas aeruginosa* infections." *Microbiology* 151 (12): 3873–3880.

38. Ashraf, R., R. A. Khan, and I. Ashraf. 2011. "Garlic (*Allium sativum*) supplementation with standard antidiabetic agent provides better diabetic control in type 2 diabetes patients." *Pakistan Journal of Pharmaceutical Sciences* 24 (4): 565–570.

39. Mix, Charles, Bernard Fantus, and William Augustus Evans. *The Practical Medicine Series*. Chicago, Illinois: The Year Book Publishers, 1918.

40. Sasaki, J., T. Kita, K. Ishita, H. Uchisawa, and H. Matsue. 1999. "Antibacterial activity of garlic powder against *Escherichia coli* O-157." *Journal of Nutritional Science and Vitaminology* (Tokyo) 45: 785–790.

41. Ushimaru, P. I., L. N. Barbosa, A. A. Fernandes, L. C. Di Stasi, and A. Fernandes Jr. 2012. "*In vitro* antibacterial activity of medicinal plant extracts against *Escherichia coli* strains from human clinical specimens and interactions with antimicrobial drugs." *Natural Products Research* 26 (16): 1553–1557.

42. Palaksha, M. N., M. Ahmed, and S. Das. 2010. "Antibacterial activity of garlic extract on streptomycin-resistant *Staphylococcus aureus* and *Escherichia coli* solely and in synergism with streptomycin." *Journal of Natural Science Biology and Medicine* 1 (1): 12–15.

43. Kaschula, C. H., R. Hunter, J. Cotton, R. Tuveri, E. Ngarande, K. Dzobo, G. Schäfer, V. Siyo, D. Lang, D. A. Kusza, B. Davies, A. A. Katz, and M. I. Parker. 2016. "The garlic compound ajoene targets protein folding in the endoplasmic reticulum of cancer cells." *Molecular Carcinogenesis* 55 (8): 1213–1228.

44. Yin, X., R. Zhang, C. Feng, J. Zhang, D. Liu, K. Xu, X. Wang, S. Zhang, Z. Li, X. Liu, and H. Ma. 2014. "Diallyl disulfide induces G2/M arrest and promotes apoptosis through the p53/p21 and MEK-ERK pathways in human esophageal squamous cell carcinoma." *Oncology Reports* 32 (4): 1748–1756.

45. Kodali, R. T., and G. D. Eslick. 2015. "Meta-analysis: Does garlic intake reduce risk of gastric cancer?" *Nutritional Cancer* 67 (1): 1–11.

46. Gonzalez, C. A., G. Pera, A. Agudo, H. B. Bueno-de-Mesquita, M. Ceroti, H. Boeing, M. Schulz, G. Del Giudice, M. Plebani, F. Carneiro, F. Berrino, C. Sacerdote, R. Tumino, S. Panico, G. Berglund, H. Siman, G. Hallmans, R. Stenling, C. Martinez, M. Dorronsoro, A. Barricarte, C. Navarro, J. R. Quiros, N. Allen, T. J. Key, S. Bingham, N. E. Day, J. Linseisen, G. Nagel, K. Overvad, M. K. Jensen, A. Olsen, A. Tjonneland, F. L. Buchner, P. H. Peeters, M. E. Numans, F. Clavel-Chapelon, M. C. Boutron-Ruault, D. Roukos,

A. Trichopoulou, T. Psaltopoulou, E. Lund, C. Casagrande, N. Slimani, M. Jenab, and E. Riboli. 2006. "Fruit and vegetable intake and the risk of stomach and oesophagus adenocarcinoma in the European Prospective Investigation into Cancer and Nutrition (EPIC-EURGAST)." *International Journal of Cancer* 118: 2559–2566.

47. Zhang, W., M. Ha, Y. Gong, Y. Xu, N. Dong, and Y. Yuan. 2010. "Allicin induces apoptosis in gastric cancer cells through activation of both extrinsic and intrinsic pathways." *Oncology Reports* 24: 1585–1592.

48. Yan, J. Y., F. M. Tian, W. N. Hu, J. H. Zhang, H. F. Cai, and N. Li. 2013. "Apoptosis of human gastric cancer cells line SGC 7901 induced by garlic-derived compound S-allylmercaptocysteine (SAMC)." *European Review for Medical and Pharmacological Sciences* 17 (6): 745–751.

49. Park, H. S., G. Y. Kim, I. W. Choi, N. D. Kim, H. J. Hwang, Y. W. Choi, and Y. H. Choi. 2011. "Inhibition of matrix metalloproteinase activities and tightening of tight junctions by diallyl disulfide in AGS human gastric carcinoma cells." *Journal of Food Science* 76: T105–111.

50. Park, E. Y., S. H. Ki, M. S. Ko, C. W. Kim, M. H. Lee, Y. S. Lee, and S. G. Kim. 2005. "Garlic oil and DDB, comprised in a pharmaceutical composition for the treatment of patients with viral hepatitis, prevents acute liver injuries potentiated by glutathione deficiency in rats." *Chemical Biological Interactions* 155 (1–2): 82–96.

51. Lee, M. H., Kim, Y. M., and Kim, S. G. 2012. "Efficacy and tolerability of diphenyl-dimethyl-dicarboxylate plus garlic oil in patients with chronic hepatitis." *International Journal of Clinical Pharmacology and Therapeutics* 50 (11): 778–786.

52. Xiong, X. J., Wang, P. Q., Li, S. J., Li, X. K., Zhang, Y. Q., and Wang, J. 2015. "Garlic for hypertension: A systematic review and meta-analysis of randomized controlled trials." *Phytomedicine* 22 (3): 352–361.

53. Ried, K., O. R. Frank, and N. P. Stocks. 2013. "Aged garlic extract reduces blood pressure in hypertensives: a dose–response trial." *European Journal of Clinical Nutrition* 67 (1): 64–70.

54. Ried, K., N. Travica, and A. Sali. 2016. "The effect of aged garlic extract on blood pressure and other cardiovascular risk factors in uncontrolled hypertensives: the AGE at heart trial." *Integrated Blood Pressure Control* 9: 9–21.

55. Mahdavi-Roshan, M., J. Nasrollahzadeh, A. Mohammad Zadeh, and A. Zahedmehr. 2016. "Does garlic supplementation control blood pressure in patients with severe coronary artery disease? A clinical trial study." *Iranian Red Crescent Medical Journal* 18 (11): e23871.

56. Bordia, A., S. K. Verma, and K. C. Srivastava. 1998. "Effect of garlic (*Allium sativum*) on blood lipids, blood sugar, fibrinogen and fibrinolytic activity in patients with coronary artery disease." *Prostaglandins, Leukotrienes, & Essential Fatty Acids* 58: 257–263.

57. Ashraf, R., et al., "Garlic (*Allium sativum*) supplementation with standard anti-diabetic agent provides better diabetic control in type 2 diabetes patients."

58. Ledezma, E., J. C. López, P. Marin, H. Romero, G. Ferrara, L. De Sousa, A. Jorquera, and R. Apitz Castro. 1999. "Ajoene in the topical short-term treatment of tinea cruris and tinea corporis in humans. Randomized comparative study with terbinafine." *Arzneimittelforschung* 49 (6): 544–547.

59. Kianoush, S., M. Balali-Mood, S. R. Mousavi, V. Moradi, M. Sadeghi, B. Dadpour, O. Rajabi, and M. T. Shakeri. 2012. "Comparison of therapeutic effects of garlic and d-Penicillamine in patients with chronic occupational lead poisoning." *Basic & Clinical Pharmacology & Toxicology* 110 (5): 476–481.

60. Jeong, J. W., S. Park, C. Park, Y. C. Chang, D. O. Moon, S. O. Kim, G. Y. Kim, H. J. Cha, H. S. Kim, Y. W. Choi, W. J. Kim, Y. H. Yoo, and Y. H. Choi. 2014. "N-benzyl-N-methyldecan-1-amine, a phenylamine derivative isolated from garlic cloves, induces G2/M phase arrest and apoptosis in U937 human leukemia cells." *Oncology Reports* 32 (1): 373–381.

61. Park C., S. Park, Y. H. Chung, G. Y. Kim, Y. W. Choi, B. W. Kim, and Y. H. Choi. 2014. "Induction of apoptosis by a hexane extract of aged black garlic in the human leukemic U937 cells." *Nutritional Research and Practice* 8 (2): 132–137.

62. Ling H., J. He, H. Tan, L. Yi, F. Liu, X. Ji, Y. Wu, H. Hu, X. Zeng, X. Ai, H. Jiang, and Q. Su. 2017. "Identification of potential targets for differentiation in human leukemia cells induced by diallyl disulfide." *International Journal of Oncology* 50 (2): 697–707.

63. Xu, B., B. Monsarrat, J. E. Gairin, and E. Girbal-Neuhauser. 2004. "Effect of ajoene, a natural antitumor small molecule, on human 20S proteasome activity in vitro and in human leukemic HL60 cells." *Fundamentals of Clinical Pharmacology* 18 (2): 171–180.

64. Linares, M. B., M. D. Garrido, C. Martins, and L. Patarata. 2013. "Efficacies of garlic and *L. sakei* in wine-based marinades for controlling *Listeria monocytogenes* and *Salmonella* spp. in *chouriço de vinho*, a dry sausage made from wine-marinated pork." *Journal of Food Science* 78 (5): 719–724.

65. Myneni, A. A., S. C. Chang, R. Niu, L. Liu, M. K. Swanson, J. Li, J. Su, G. A. Giovino, S. Yu, Z. F. Zhang, and L. Mu. 2016. "Raw garlic consumption and lung cancer in a Chinese population." *Cancer Epidemiology, Biomarkers & Prevention* 25 (4): 624–633.

66. Wang, Y., Z. Sun, S. Chen, Y. Jiao, and C. Bai. 2016. "ROS-mediated activation of JNK/p38 contributes partially to the pro-apoptotic effect of ajoene on cells of lung adenocarcinoma." *Tumour Biology* 37 (3): 3727–3738.

67. Wang, K., Y. Wang, Q. Qi, F. Zhang, Y. Zhang, X. Zhu, G. Liu, Y. Luan, Z. Zhao, J. Cai, J. Cao, and S. Li. 2016. "Inhibitory effects of S-allylmercaptocysteine against benzo(a)pyrene-induced precancerous carcinogenesis in human lung cells." *International Immunopharmacology* 34: 37–43.

68. Coppi, A., M. Cabinian, D. Mirelman, and P. Sinnis. 2006. "Antimalarial activity of allicin, a biologically active compound from garlic cloves." *Antimicrobial Agents and Chemotherapy* 50 (5): 1731–1737.

69. Mishra, S. K., O. P. Asthana, S. Mohanty, J. K. Patnaik, B. S. Das, J. S. Srivastava, S. K. Satpathy, S. Dash, P. K. Rath, and K. Varghese. 1995. "Effectiveness of α, β-arteether in acute falciparum malaria." *Transactions of the Royal Society of Tropical Medicine and Hygiene* 89 (3): 299–301.

70. Govindan, V., A. N. Panduranga, and P. Krishna Murthy. 2016. "Assessment of in vivo antimalarial activity of arteether and garlic oil combination therapy." *Biochemistry and Biophysics Reports* 5: 359–364.

71. Wang, Q., Y. Wang, Z. Ji, X. Chen, Y. Pan, G. Gao, H. Gu, Y. Yang, B. C. Choi, and Y. Yan. 2012. "Risk factors for multiple myeloma: a hospital-based case-control study in Northwest China." *Cancer Epidemiology* 36 (5): 439–444.

72. Shams-Ghahfarokhi, M., M. R. Shokoohamiri, N. Amirrajab, B. Moghadasi, A. Ghajari, F. Zeini, G. Sadeghi, and M. Razzaghi-Abyaneh. 2006. "In vitro antifungal activities of *Allium cepa*, *Allium sativum* and ketoconazole against some pathogenic yeasts and dermatophytes." *Fitoterapia* 77 (4): 321–323.

73. Li, W. R., Q. S. Shi, H. Q. Dai, Q. Liang, X. B. Xie, X. M. Huang, G. Z. Zhao, and L. X. Zhang. 2016. "Antifungal activity, kinetics and molecular mechanism of action of garlic oil against *Candida albicans*." *Science Reports* 6: 22805.

74. Lee, H. S., C. H. Lee, H. C. Tsai, and D. M. Salter. 2009. "Inhibition of cyclo-oxygenase 2 expression by diallyl sulfide on joint inflammation induced by urate crystal and IL-1beta." *Osteoarthritis Cartilage* 17 (1): 91–99.

75. Williams, F. M., J. Skinner, T. D. Spector, A. Cassidy, I. M. Clark, R. M. Davidson, and A. J. MacGregor. 2010. "Dietary garlic and hip osteoarthritis: evidence of a protective effect and putative mechanism of action." *BMC Musculoskeletal Disorders* 11: 280.

76. Mukherjee, M., A. S. Das, S. Mitra, and C. Mitra. 2004. "Prevention of bone loss by oil extract of garlic (*Allium sativum* Linn.) in an ovariectomized rat model of osteoporosis." *Phytotherapy Research* 18 (5): 389–394.

77. Mukherjee, M., A. S. Das, D. Das, S. Mukherjee, S. Mitra, and C. Mitra. 2006. "Role of oil extract of garlic (*Allium sativum* Linn.) on intestinal transference of calcium and its possible correlation with preservation of skeletal health

in an ovariectomized rat model of osteoporosis." *Phytotherapy Research* 20 (5): 408–415.

78. Mukherjee, M., A. S. Das, D. Das, S. Mukherjee, S. Mitra, and C. Mitra. 2006. "Effects of garlic oil on postmenopausal osteoporosis using ovariectomized rats: comparison with the effects of lovastatin and 17beta-estradiol." *Phytotherapy Research* 20 (1): 21–27.

79. Bagul, M., S. Kakumanu, and T. A. Wilson. 2015. "Crude garlic extract inhibits cell proliferation and induces cell cycle arrest and apoptosis of cancer cells in vitro." *Journal of Medicinal Food* 18 (7): 731–737.

80. Zhou, X. F., Z. S. Ding, and N. B. Liu. 2013. "Allium vegetables and risk of prostate cancer: evidence from 132,192 subjects." *Asian Pacific Journal of Cancer Prevention* 14 (7): 4131–4134.

81. Sigounas, G., J. Hooker, A. Anagnostou, and M. Steiner. 1997. "S-allylmercaptocysteine inhibits cell proliferation and reduces the viability of erythroleukemia, breast, and prostate cancer cell lines." *Nutrition and Cancer* 27: 186–191.

82. Denisov, L. N., I. V. Andrianova, and S. S. Timofeeva. 1999. "Garlic effectiveness in rheumatoid arthritis." *Terapevticheskii Arkhiv* 71 (8): 55–58.

83. Ahmed, W., A. Zaki, and T. Nabil. 2015. "Prevention of methotrexate-induced nephrotoxicity by concomitant administration of garlic aqueous extract in rat." *Turkish Journal of Medicinal Sciences* 45 (3): 507–516.

84. Ledezma, E., et al., "Ajoene in the topical short-term treatment of tinea cruris and tinea corporis in humans."

85. Eja, M. E., B. E. Asikong, C. Abriba, G. E. Arikpo, E. E. Anwan, and K. H. Enyi-Idoh. 2007. "A comparative assessment of the antimicrobial effects of garlic (*Allium sativum*) and antibiotics on diarrheagenic organisms." *Southeast Asian Journal of Tropical Medicine and Public Health* 38 (2): 343–348.

86. Linares, M. B., et al., "Efficacies of garlic and *L. sakei* in wine-based marinades for controlling *Listeria monocytogenes* and *Salmonella* spp. in *chouriço de vinho*, a dry sausage made from wine-marinated pork."

87. Rapp, A., G. Grohmann, P. Oelzner, B. Uehleke, and C. Uhlemann. 2006. "Does garlic influence rheologic properties and blood flow in progressive systemic sclerosis?" *Forschende Komplementärmedizin* 13 (3): 141–146.

88. Sasaki, J., T. Kita, K. Ishita, H. Uchisawa, H. Matsue. 1999. "Antibacterial activity of garlic powder against *Escherichia coli* O-157." *Journal of Nutritional Science and Vitaminology* 45 (6): 785–790.

89. Naganawa, R., N. Iwata, K. Ishikawa, H. Fukuda, T. Fujino, and A. Suzuki. 1996. "Inhibition of microbial growth by ajoene, a sulfur-containing compound derived from garlic." *Applied and Environmental Microbiology* 62 (11): 4238–4242.

90. Mozaffari Nejad, A. S., S. Shabani, M. Bayat, and S. E. Hosseini. 2014. "Antibacterial effect of garlic aqueous extract on *Staphylococcus aureus* in hamburger." *Jundishapur Journal of Microbiology* 7 (11): e13134.

91. Sabitha, P., P. M. Adhikari, S. M. Shenoy, A. Kamath, R. John, M. V. Prabhu, S. Mohammed, S. Baliga, and U. Padmaja. 2005. "Efficacy of garlic paste in oral candidiasis." *Tropical Doctor* 35 (2): 99–100.

92. Jain, R. C. 1998. "Anti tubercular activity of garlic oil." *Indian Journal of Pathology and Microbiology* 41 (1): 131.

93. Hasan, N., N. Yusuf, Z. Toossi, and N. Islam. 2006. "Suppression of *Mycobacterium tuberculosis* induced reactive oxygen species (ROS) and TNF-alpha mRNA expression in human monocytes by allicin." FEBS Letters 580 (10): 2517–2522.

94. Hannan, A., M. Ikram Ullah, M. Usman, S. Hussain, M. Absar, and K. Javed. 2011. "Anti-mycobacterial activity of garlic (*Allium sativum*) against multi-drug resistant and non-multi-drug resistant *Mycobacterium tuberculosis*." *Pakistan Journal of Pharmaceutical Sciences* 24 (1): 81–85.

95. Balaha, M., S. Kandeel, and W. Elwan. 2016. "Garlic oil inhibits dextran sodium sulfate-induced ulcerative colitis in rats." *Life Sciences* 146: 40–51.

96. Shi, L., Q. Lin, X. Li, Y. Nie, S. Sun, X. Deng, L. Wang, J. Lu, Y. Tang, and F. Luo. 2017. "Alliin, a garlic organosulfur compound, ameliorates gut inflammation through MAPK-NF-κB/AP-1/STAT-1 inactivation and PPAR-γ activation." *Molecular Nutrition and Food Research* 61 (9).

97. Ibrahim, A. N. 2013. "Comparison of in vitro activity of metronidazole and garlic-based product (Tomex®) on *Trichomonas vaginalis*." *Parasitology Research*. 112 (5): 2063–2067.

98. Ebrahimy, F., M. Dolatian, F. Moatar, and H. A. Majd. 2015. "Comparison of the therapeutic effects of Garcin® and fluconazole on *Candida* vaginitis." *Singapore Medical Journal* 56 (10): 567–572.

99. Kim, H. K. 2016. "Garlic supplementation ameliorates UV-induced photoaging in hairless mice by regulating antioxidative activity and MMPs expression." *Molecules* 21 (1): 70.

100. Imai, J., N. Ide, Nagae S, T. Moriguchi, H. Matsuura, and Y. Itakura. 1994. "Antioxidant and radical scavenging effects of aged garlic extract and its constituents." *Planta Medica* 60: 417–420.

101. Li, G., Z. Shi, H. Jia, J. Ju, X. Wang, Z. Xia, L. Qin, C. Ge, Y. Xu, L. Cheng, P. Chen, and G. Yuan. 2000. "A clinical investigation on garlicin injectio for treatment of unstable angina pectoris and its actions on plasma endothelin and blood sugar levels." *Journal of Traditional Chinese Medicine* 20 (4): 243–246.

102. Rahman, K., and D. Billington. 2000. "Dietary supplementation with aged garlic extract inhibits ADP-induced platelet aggregation in humans." *Journal of Nutrition* 130: 2662–2665.

103. Bordia, A., et al., "Effect of garlic (*Allium sativum*) on blood lipids, blood sugar, fibrinogen and fibrinolytic activity in patients with coronary artery disease."

104. Thomas, A., S. Thakur, and S. Mhambrey. 2015. "Comparison of the anti-microbial efficacy of chlorhexidine, sodium fluoride, fluoride with essential oils, alum, green tea, and garlic with lime mouth rinses on cariogenic microbes." *Journal of International Society of Preventative and Community Dentistry* 5 (4): 302–308.

105. Fani, M. M., J. Kohanteb, and M. Dayaghi. 2007. "Inhibitory activity of garlic (*Allium sativum*) extract on multidrug-resistant *Streptococcus mutans*." *Journal of Indian Society of Pedodontics and Preventative Dentistry* 25 (4): 164–168.

106. White, E., and Sherlock, C. 2005. "The effect of nutritional therapy for yeast infection (candidiasis) in cases of chronic fatigue syndrome." *Journal of Orthomolecular Medicine* 20 (3): 193–209.

107. Yousuf, S., et al., "Effect of diallyldisulphide on an antioxidant enzyme system in *Candida* species."

108. Mukherjee, D., and S. Banerjee. 2013. "Learning and memory promoting effects of crude garlic extract." *Indian Journal of Experimental Biology* 51 (12): 1094–1100.

109. Pintana, H., J. Sripetchwandee, L. Supakul, N. Apaijai, N. Chattipakorn, and S. Chattipakorn. 2014. "Garlic extract attenuates brain mitochondrial dysfunction and cognitive deficit in obese-insulin resistant rats." *Applied Physiology, Nutrition and Metabolism* 39 (12): 1373–1379.

110. Ghasemi, S., M. Hosseini, A. Feizpour, F. Alipour, A. Sadeghi, F. Vafaee, T. Mohammadpour, M. Soukhtanloo, A. Ebrahimzadeh Bideskan, and F. Beheshti. 2017. "Beneficial effects of garlic on learning and memory deficits and brain tissue damages induced by lead exposure during juvenile rat growth is comparable to the effect of ascorbic acid." *Drug and Chemical Toxicology* 40 (2): 206–214.

111. Weber, N. D., D. O. Andersen, J. A. North, B. K. Murray, L. D. Lawson, and B. G. Hughes. 1992. "In vitro virucidal effects of *Allium sativum* (garlic) extract and compounds." *Planta Medica* 58: 417–423.

112. Nantz, M. P., C. A. Rowe, C. E. Muller, R. A. Creasy, J. M. Stanilka, and S. S. Percival. 2012. "Supplementation with aged garlic extract improves both NK and γδ-T cell function and reduces the severity of cold and flu symptoms:

a randomized, double-blind, placebo-controlled nutrition intervention." *Clinical Nutrition* 31 (3): 337–344.

113. Josling P., "Preventing the common cold with a garlic supplement: a double-blind, placebo-controlled survey."

114. Dehghani, F., A. Merat, M. R. Panjehshahin, and F. Handjani. 2005. "Healing effect of garlic extract on warts and corns." *International Journal of Dermatology* 44: 612–615.

115. Bielory, L. 2004. "Complementary and alternative interventions in asthma, allergy, and immunology." *Annals of Allergy, Asthma & Immunology* 93 (2 Suppl 1): S45–54.

116. Shams-Ghahfarokhi, M., et al., "In vitro antifungal activities of *Allium cepa*, *Allium sativum* and ketoconazole against some pathogenic yeasts and dermatophytes."

117. Bakhshi, M., J. B. Taheri, S. B. Shabestari, A. Tanik, and R. Pahlevan. 2012. "Comparison of therapeutic effect of aqueous extract of garlic and nystatin mouthwash in denture stomatitis." *Gerodontology* 29 (2): e680–684.

118. Mendoza-Juache, A., S. Aranda-Romo, J. R. Bermeo-Escalona, A. Gómez-Hernández, A. Pozos-Guillén, and L. O. Sánchez-Vargas. 2017. "The essential oil of *Allium sativum* as an alternative agent against *Candida* isolated from dental prostheses." *Revista Iberoamericana de Micología* 34 (3): 158–164.

119. Eja, M. E., B. E. Asikong, C. Abriba, G. E. Arikpo, E. E. Anwan, and K. H. Enyi-Idoh. 2007. "A comparative assessment of the antimicrobial effects of garlic (*Allium sativum*) and antibiotics on diarrheagenic organisms." *Southeast Asian Journal of Tropical Medicine and Public Health* 38 (2): 343–348.

120. Pantoja, C. V., L. C. Chiang, B. C. Norris, and J. B. Concha. 1991. "Diuretic, natriuretic and hypotensive effects produced by *Allium sativum* (garlic) in anaesthetized dogs." *Journal of Ethnopharmacology* 31 (3): 325–331.

121. Galeone, C., C. Pelucchi, R. Talamini, E. Negri, L. Dal Maso, M. Montella, V. Ramazzotti, S. Franceschi, and C. La Vecchia. 2007. "Onion and garlic intake and the odds of benign prostatic hyperplasia." *Urology* 70 (4): 672–676.

122. Chung, K. S., S. J. Shin, N. Y. Lee, S. Y. Cheon, W. Park, S. H. Sun, and H. J. An. 2016. "Anti-proliferation effects of garlic (*Allium sativum* L.) on the progression of benign prostatic hyperplasia." *Phytotherapy Research* 30 (7): 1197–1203.

123. Su, Q. S., Y. Tian, J. G. Zhang, and H. Zhang. 2008. "Effects of allicin supplementation on plasma markers of exercise-induced muscle damage, IL-6 and antioxidant capacity." *European Journal of Applied Physiology* 103 (3): 275–283.

124. Womack, C. J., D. J. Lawton, L. Redmond, M. K. Todd, and T. A. Hargens. 2015. "The effects of acute garlic supplementation on the fibrinolytic and

vasoreactive response to exercise." *Journal of the International Society of Sports Nutrition* 12: 23.

125. Clement, Y. N., J. Morton-Gittens, L. Basdeo, A. Blades, M. J. Francis, N. Gomes, M. Janjua, and A. Singh. 2007. "Perceived efficacy of herbal remedies by users accessing primary healthcare in Trinidad." *BMC Complementary and Alternative Medicine* 7: 4.

126. Liu, Y., T. M. Che, M. Song, J. J. Lee, J. A. Almeida, D. Bravo, W. G. Van Alstine, and J. E. Pettigrew. 2013. "Dietary plant extracts improve immune responses and growth efficiency of pigs experimentally infected with porcine reproductive and respiratory syndrome virus." *Journal of Animal Science* 91 (12): 5668–5679.

127. Percival, S. S. 2016. "Aged garlic extract modifies human immunity." *Journal of Nutrition* 146 (2): 433S–436S.

128. Ibid.

129. Miean, K. H., and S. Mohamed. 2001. "Flavonoid (myricetin, quercetin, kaempferol, luteolin, and apigenin) content of edible tropical plants." *Journal of Agriculture and Food Chemistry* 49 (6): 3106–3112.

130. Marschollek, C., F. Karimzadeh, M. Jafarian, M. Ahmadi, S. M. Mohajeri, S. Rahimi, E. J. Speckmann, and A. Gorji. 2017. "Effects of garlic extract on spreading depression: *In vitro* and *in vivo* investigations." *Nutritional Neuroscience* 20 (2): 127–134.

131. Kianoush, S., et al., "Comparison of therapeutic effects of garlic and d-Penicillamine in patients with chronic occupational lead poisoning."

132. Xiong, X. J., et al., "Garlic for hypertension: A systematic review and meta-analysis of randomized controlled trials."

133. Ko, J. W., J. Y. Shin, J. W. Kim, S. H. Park, N. R. Shin, I. C. Lee, I. S. Shin, C. Moon, S. H. Kim, S. H. Kim, and J. C. Kim. 2017. "Protective effects of diallyl disulfide against acetaminophen-induced nephrotoxicity: A possible role of CYP2E1 and NF-κB." *Food and Chemical Toxicology* 102: 156–165.

134. Sumioka, I., T. Matsura, and K. Yamada. 2001. "Therapeutic effect of S-allylmercaptocysteine on acetaminophen-induced liver injury in mice." *European Journal of Pharmacology* 433: 177–185.

135. Naji, K. M., E. S. Al-Shaibani, F. A. Alhadi, S. A. Al-Soudi, and M. R. D'souza. 2017. "Hepatoprotective and antioxidant effects of single clove garlic against CCl4-induced hepatic damage in rabbits." *BMC Complementary and Alternative Medicine* 17 (1): 411.

136. Park, E. Y., et al., "Garlic oil and DDB, comprised in a pharmaceutical composition for the treatment of patients with viral hepatitis, prevents acute liver injuries potentiated by glutathione deficiency in rats."

137. Bespalov, V. G., et al., "Study of an antioxidant dietary supplement 'Karinat' in patients with benign breast disease."

138. Lee, E. K., S. W. Chung, J. Y. Kim, J. M. Kim, H. S. Heo, H. A. Lim, M. K. Kim, S. Anton, T. Yokozawa, and H. Y. Chung. 2009. "Allylmethylsulfide down-regulates X-ray irradiation-induced nuclear factor-kappaB signaling in C57/BL6 mouse kidney." *Journal of Medicine and Food* 12 (3): 542–551.

139. Chang, H. S., D. Endoh, Y. Ishida, H. Takahashi, S. Ozawa, M. Hayashi, A. Yabuki, and O. Yamato. 2012. "Radioprotective effect of alk(en)yl thiosulfates derived from allium vegetables against DNA damage caused by X-ray irradiation in cultured cells: antiradiation potential of onions and garlic." *The Scientific World Journal* 2012: 846750.

140. Abrams, G. A., and M. B. Fallon. 1998. "Treatment of hepatopulmonary syndrome with *Allium sativum* L. (garlic): a pilot trial." *Journal of Clinical Gastroenterology* 27 (3): 232–235.

141. Najafi Sani, M., H. R. Kianifar, A. Kianee, and G. Khatami. 2006. "Effect of oral garlic on arterial oxygen pressure in children with hepatopulmonary syndrome." *World Journal of Gastroenterology* 12 (15): 2427–2431.

142. O'Gara, E. A., D. J. Hill, and D. J. Maslin. 2000. "Activities of garlic oil, garlic powder, and their diallyl constituents against *Helicobacter pylori*." *Applied and Environmental Microbiology* 66: 2269–73.

143. Sivam, G. P. 2001. "Protection against *Helicobacter pylori* and other bacterial infections by garlic." *Journal of Nutrition* 131 (3s): 1106S–1108S.

144. Jonkers, D., E. van den Broek, I. van Dooren, C. Thijs, E. Dorant, G. Hageman, and E. Stobberingh. 1999. "Antibacterial effect of garlic and omeprazole on *Helicobacter pylori*." *The Journal of Antimicrobial Chemotherapy* 43 (6): 837–839.

145. El-Ashmawy, N. E., E. G. Khedr, H. A. El-Bahrawy, and H. M. Selim. 2016. "Gastroprotective effect of garlic in indomethacin induced gastric ulcer in rats." *Nutrition* 32 (7–8): 849–854.

146. Pai, S. T., and M. W. Platt. 1995. "Antifungal effects of *Allium sativum* (garlic) extract against the *Aspergillus* species involved in otomycosis." *Letters in Applied Microbiology* 20 (1): 14–18.

147. Kenawy, S., G. F. Mohammed, S. Younes, and A. I. Elakhras. 2014. "Evaluation of TNF-α serum level in patients with recalcitrant multiple common warts, treated by lipid garlic extract." *Dermatologic Therapy* 27 (5): 272–277.

148. Oi, Y., T. Kawada, C. Shishido, K. Wada, Y. Kominato, S. Nishimura, T. Ariga, and K. Iwai. 1999. "Allyl-containing sulfides in garlic increase uncoupling protein content in brown adipose tissue, and noradrenaline and adrenaline secretion in rats." *Journal of Nutrition* 129 (2): 336–342.

149. Soleimani, D., Z. Paknahad, G. Askari, B. Iraj, and A. Feizi. 2016. "Effect of garlic powder consumption on body composition in patients with nonalcoholic fatty liver disease: A randomized, double-blind, placebo-controlled trial." *Advanced Biomedical Research* 5: 2.

150. Ejaz, S., I. Chekarova, J. W. Cho, S. Y. Lee, S. Ashraf, and C. W. Lim. 2009. "Effect of aged garlic extract on wound healing: a new frontier in wound management." *Drug and Chemical Toxicology* 32 (3): 191–203.

151. Sarhan, W. A., H. M. Azzazy, and I. M. El-Sherbiny. 2016. "Honey/chitosan nanofiber wound dressing enriched with *Allium sativum* and *Cleome droserifolia*: enhanced antimicrobial and wound healing activity." *ACS Applied Materials & Interfaces* 8 (10): 6379–6390.

152. Palacio-Landín, J., P. Mendoza-de Gives, D. O. Salinas-Sánchez, M. E. López-Arellano, E. Liébano-Hernández, V. M. Hernández-Velázquez, and M. G. Valladares-Cisneros. 2015. "*In vitro* and *in vivo* nematocidal activity of *Allium sativum* and *Tagetes erecta* extracts against *Haemonchus contortus*." *Turkiye Parazitolojii Dergisi* 39 (4): 260–264.

153. Plata-Rueda, A., L. C. Martínez, M. H. D. Santos, F. L. Fernandes, C. F. Wilcken, M. A. Soares, J. E. Serrão, and J. C. Zanuncio. 2017. "Insecticidal activity of garlic essential oil and their constituents against the mealworm beetle, *Tenebrio molitor* Linnaeus (Coleoptera: Tenebrionidae)." *Scientific Reports* 7: 46406.

154. Wang, X., Q. Li, L. Shen, J. Yang, H. Cheng, S. Jiang, C. Jiang, and H. Wang. 2014. "Fumigant, contact, and repellent activities of essential oils against the darkling beetle, *Alphitobius diaperinus*." *Journal of Insect Science* 14: 75.

155. Hile, A. G., Z. Shan, S. Z. Zhang, and E. Block. 2004. "Aversion of European starlings (*Sturnus vulgaris*) to garlic oil treated granules: garlic oil as an avian repellent. Garlic oil analysis by nuclear magnetic resonance spectroscopy." *Journal of Agriculture and Food Chemistry* 52 (8): 2192–2196.

156. Qualls, W. A., J. Scott-Fiorenzano, G. C. Müller, K. L. Arheart, J. C. Beier, and R. D. Xue. 2016. "Evaluation and adaptation of attractive toxic sugar baits for *Culex tarsalis* and *Culex quinquefasciatus* control in the Coachella Valley, Southern California." *The American Mosquito Control Association* 32 (4): 292–299.

157. Junnila, A., E. E. Revay, G. C. Müller, V. Kravchenko, W. A. Qualls, R. D. Xue, S. A. Allen, J. C. Beier, and Y. Schlein. 2015. "Efficacy of attractive toxic sugar baits (ATSB) against *Aedes albopictus* with garlic oil encapsulated in beta-cyclodextrin (sugar) as the active ingredient." *Acta Tropica* 152: 195–200.

158. Garrett, H., J. Ferguson, and M. Amaranthus. 2012. *Organic Management for the Professional*. Austin, Texas: University of Texas Press.

159. Hata, F. T., M. U. Ventura, M. G. Carvalho, A. L. Miguel, M. S. Souza, M. T. Paula, and M. A. Zawadneak. 2016. "Intercropping garlic plants reduces *Tetranychus urticae* in strawberry crop." *Experimental and Applied Acarology* 69 (3): 311–321.

160. Rahimi-Esboei, B., M. A. Ebrahimzadeh, H. Fathi, and F. Rezaei Anzahaei. 2016. "Scolicidal effect of *Allium sativum* flowers on hydatid cyst protoscolices." *The European Review for Medical and Pharmacological Sciences* 20 (1): 129–132.

161. Bharadwaj, A., L. E. Hayes, and K. C. Stafford. 2015. "Effectiveness of garlic for the control of *Ixodes scapularis* (Acari: Ixodidae) on residential properties in Western Connecticut." *Journal of Medical Entomology* 52 (4): 722–725.

162. Mirondo, Rita, et al., "Deodorization of garlic breath by foods, and the role of polyphenol oxidase and phenolic compounds."

163. Koscielny, J., D. Klüssendorf, R. Latza, R. Schmitt, H. Radtke, G. Siegel, H. Kiesewetter. 1999. "The antiatherosclerotic effect of *Allium sativum*." *Atherosclerosis* 144 (1): 237–249.

164. Xiong, X. J., P. Q. Wang, S. J. Li, X. K. Li, Y. Q. Zhang, J. Wang. 2015. "Garlic for hypertension: A systematic review and meta-analysis of randomized controlled trials." *Phytomedicine* 22 (3): 352–361. doi:10.1016/j.phymed.2014.12.013

165. Bonaduce, I., M. P. Colombini, and S. Diring. 2006. "Identification of garlic in old gildings by gas chromatography–mass spectrometry." *Journal of Chromatography A* 1107 (1–2): 226–232.

ABOUT THE AUTHOR

SUSAN BRANSON earned an undergraduate degree in biology from St. Francis Xavier University, then a MSc in toxicology from the University of Ottawa. From there, she worked in research: in the field, in the lab, as a writer, and as an administrator. She took time off and stayed at home after her second child was born. In addition to being a stay-at-home mom, she also took violin lessons, photography courses, earned a diploma in writing, and ultimately became a holistic nutritional consultant. Susan is a member of CSNN's Alumni Association, Canada's leading holistic nutrition school.

ABOUT FAMILIUS

VISIT OUR WEBSITE: WWW.FAMILIUS.COM
JOIN OUR FAMILY

There are lots of ways to connect with us! Subscribe to our newsletters at www.familius.com to receive uplifting daily inspiration, essays from our Pater Familius, a free ebook every month, and the first word on special discounts and Familius news.

GET BULK DISCOUNTS

If you feel a few friends and family might benefit from what you've read, let us know and we'll be happy to provide you with quantity discounts. Simply email us at orders@familius.com.

CONNECT

Facebook: www.facebook.com/paterfamilius
Twitter: @familiustalk, @paterfamilius1
Pinterest: www.pinterest.com/familius
Instagram: @familiustalk

FAMILIUS

THE MOST IMPORTANT WORK YOU
EVER DO WILL BE WITHIN THE
WALLS OF YOUR OWN HOME.

CPSIA information can be obtained
at www.ICGtesting.com
Printed in the USA
FSHW04n0934080318
45446FS